I0462136

ADHD is not a Sentence

ADHD IS NOT A SENTENCE

My life travels that led me to medicine
and a full and comprehensive understanding of ADHD

DR ROBERT GARSIA

©2014 Dr. Robert Garsia
All rights reserved

This book is a work of non-fiction

Book formatting and design by www.finitepublishing.com
Book cover design by Steve Guest

ISBN 978-1500381059

DEDICATION

To my loving wife for having coped so well with me and my ADD
children; and to the parents, carers, teachers and all the patients that
have had to deal with ADD in our society.

This book has two parts. Part One deals with some of my interesting or humorous instances that I have been experienced. Part Two deals with the history, examination; including the sensory motor examination, diagnosis, treatments and prognosis of ADHD.

The motivation for this book was that so much is written about this subject and yet so much confusion and exist about a clear cut subject. I hope that I can shed a clear pathway to the proper diagnosis and treatment in our society. Confusion between just bad behaviour and a real problem does exist. Badly or untreated ADD does lead to alienation of children from our society, but a good and effective management and treatment does result in a successful outcome.

FOREWORD

I owe so much to so many people along my life's travel that I would find it very hard where to start; I sincerely hope I don't forget to some of them.

First and foremost I do owe so very much to Evelyn my wife; she did not just share my life, giving us a beautiful family and being such an asset in my practice. I need to thank all my children; that understood even when my practice took me away from family time. I must remember my brother Nelson who helped my family financially so that we could migrate to Australia. I do thank the Christian Brothers that reduced their fees for my secondary schooling; it prepared me for my career; then my training at the Melbourne University which was second to none; all my teachers at Geelong hospital in that prepared me so well for my stint in the Mission Hospital New Guinea. When I came to Brisbane, I need to thank the teachers at the Health Department the Division of Child Guidance for introducing me to Minimal Brain Dysfunction that later became know by the better name of ADHD.

I am grateful to the many pharmaceutical companies that financed seminars and educational conferences that provided further training in psychiatry by renown specialist; although many of the conferences included the better understanding of their medications that only took a minor part of the educational meeting. I would like to acknowledge the generous practitioner that took me on in Caboolture and later gave me firstly an assistantship and later a partnership.

I cannot forget to thank the many wonderful receptionists and assistant that helped me; they made such a contribution to my practice over the years. I want to thank the Education Guidance officers, school teacher and headmasters for their cooperation; they were only to willing to help children with the many problems they had. I have to be very grateful to all the patients and parents that allowed me into their lived; (and often waited a long time to see me) in several practices; both Government and private practices that I worked in. I can't forget to add how appreciative we were and that we will never forget the wonder full send off when we finally retired; we were so impressed by all of our patients-friends; past and present; that attended or sent their apologies.

CONTENTS

INTRODUCTION

I have decided to combine an autobiography of many of my experiences; some of which are funny and some that are not so funny; but they all are interesting. I will then present a synopsis of my passion as a medical practitioner; ADHD and Asperger's. I will describe the diagnosis, the management, treatment and a discussion of the subject of ADHD (and a mention of Asperger's syndrome on the way).

I was born in Egypt I came to Australia in 1952. I finished my primary school at the Pascoe Vale and I then completed secondary school at the Christian Brothers North Melbourne. I did my medical course at Melbourne University where I graduated with the degree of M.B.B.S. which is the initials of Bachelor of Medicine and Bachelor of Surgery. The training was very extensive, but it only included a very basic training in mental health. I then did two years further training as a resident doctor at the Geelong Hospital; there I got very extensive training; my training was even more thorough as the teachers there knew that I wanted to go to a mission hospital after my years at that hospital.

The extensive training in the medical specialities now seems to be wasted because most of the city hospitals require specialist degrees to be able to (practice those specialities) in order to access their beds. Then I went to a mission in New Guinea so I needed every aspect of my training. New Guinea was then called T.P.N.G (Territory of Papua New Guinea). There I needed every aspect of my training.

On my return from New Guinea to Australia; I spent several years training in mental health. I worked with a division of the Health Department. That division was then known as the Division of Child Guidance. Incidentally, the Education Department also had a division called Child Guidance. Eventually the name of our Health Department Division was changed to Child and Youth Mental Health (CYMS). The Health Department became Queensland Health. I did endeavour to do a Diploma course with the University of Queensland in mental health called a D.P.M. (Diploma of Psychiatry Mental health). I eventually, went into private practice because my financial needs grew as my family grew.

At first I started part time as a locum in a town that is called Caboolture; I later joined that practice as an associate and then was offered a partnership which accepted. I left Caboolture, after several years and started my own solo practice in an outer suburb of Brisbane called Kallangur. As I wanted to use my mental health training as well as my general practice training; so I started a general family practice so that I could treat the whole patient; without the label of a mental health clinic. The practice soon had a loading of mental health and of children with the various problems; as the word of mouth soon spread; that I was particularly interested and I was trained in mental health and child and family guidance.

I stayed in Caboolture for many years. I first moved to the now demolished Space City in Kallangur, and then moved to Good Fellows Rd. I then moved again to Anzac Ave still in Kallangur. I continued my training in mental by attending many seminars on mental health and suicide.

There I retired from my Kallangur the general practice in June 2011. My passion has always remained with the mental health of children; especially children with ADHD, ADD and Asperger's syndrome. I will take you through an account of the factors involved in ADD, factors like the genetic basis for the diagnosis, the presentation, the physical examination including the Sensory Motor examination, and many of the theoretical factors. I will discuss the many, and sometimes dramatic claims of the so called treatments for ADHD that are claimed to be successful. I will also discuss many of the myths that surround the diagnosis and treatment of ADD. I will discuss many of the reports that poo hoo traditional stimulant treatment for ADHD. I will describe the normal developmental stages; using a time frame; of the child. I will then introduce a model; that I use; to able to better understand ADHD. Finally I will discuss the management including the medication treatments options that are available for the effective treatment of ADHD and their associated condition.

PART ONE

MY LIFE

CHAPTER ONE

I don't remember much of my early years so that my recollections of my younger years are very patchy. I was born during WW2 in Alexandria, Egypt in a suburb called Embramia. I recently visited Egypt. I believe that Embramia is now a very up-market suburb, it was not when I born and lived there. I will describe what memories I do have. Then I will discuss the experiences of my recent visit.

As a child I loved sliding down the stair rail from the third floor. It was a circular staircase all the way from the third floor, so it was a really great thrill for a young child to slide the whole way down. There was a large ball at the bottom of the rail so I was always sure to come to a stop at the bottom of the long slide. However, on this particular occasion somebody had removed the stop at the end of the rail on this occasion so I kept on going. I hit my chin on the end of the rail and split it badly. As you can imagine; I started screaming as blood went everywhere. My oldest brother came to my rescue; he stopped the copious bleeding; then took me to my parents. My mother punished me for doing what I had been told not to do so many times before. Very many years later I still bear the scars on my chin, of that occasion.

I have another vague recollection; I was standing on the veranda and I was excitedly watching a bomb dropped from an air plane (I think now it was German) hit the building next door. The whole of front of the building collapsed as the bomb hit it.

I wanted to stay and watch, but my mother pulled me. I think she must have taken us away to what I now know was a bomb shelter. I guess my time was not yet up as the bomb did not hit our building and I am here to tell the story.

I think it was for my biological father's 40th birthday party; he was in Army uniform as my brother does have photographs of that occasion. He has another photo of me trying to get the last drops of wine from a Chianti bottle. I was on my head. I was four at that time. All I do recall is a party; I have another dreadful memory of the time before we left Egypt. It was during the skirmish between the Egyptians and the British; I was coming home; from school when I saw some Arabs playing football. I stopped to watch them. It was then that I realized what they were playing football with was a soldier's head. Another group had another unfortunate soldier and they were disembowelling him alive. His screams will never leave me and I do find it is very difficult to forget it. I rushed home frightened and absolutely devastated. I sometimes still recall this time in a bad dream. Thankfully those bad dreams are getting less and less these days! My surname is Garsia spelt with an S. The family has it that I my ancestors were on the wrong side of the Spanish inquisition so the left Spain and went to Portugal, so they changed their name slightly by spelling Garsia with an s instead of the usual c (Garcia). I don't think they could have been too clever, but then the authorities must not have been clever either as I am here many generations later. After I lost my biological father, my mother remarried. So my 'new' family moved to Port Said. My recollection there are a little bit better ;we lived in a roof top apartment and we kept several chooks. We had another tenant in the same building; that I recall he would say I want to go and look at your chooks now . I always wondered why he found our chooks so interesting so on day I followed him when he went out to look at the chooks; I then found out why he wanted to see the chooks; he really just wanted to pass wind! He was the musician that agreed to teach me the violin. There we stayed till we came to Australia.

We came to Australia on ship belonging to the Floata Laura line; I think it was a old transport ship. I remember many traders coming alongside the ship trying to sell their wares as we left Egypt before the Suez Canal was closed. I will later disclose what I was told as to why Egypt took over the control of the Suez Canal. This was the beginning of the trouble with the British that eventually led to Egypt taking full control of the Suez Canal. I do have some recollections of the trip to Australia. We did have a cabin on a lower deck and that the beds were quite uncomfortable. I do remember that I got terribly sea sick for the first part of the sea trip; however I must have got better as the trip went on because I don't remember being sick later on during the voyage. In those days it took the better part of a month to get to Australia. What I do remember of that journey was a party as we crossed the Equator; I must have been okay by then. It is even a tradition today that most people on board the ship are dunked in the ship's pool.

I do recall that the ship braking down when we were near the Equator. We were at anchor for a considerable time; I do recall feeling very hot then, as we had with no power for air conditioning.

I remember that we arrived at Freemantle in Australia; there was an old timber structure on the dock. All the passengers had to climb down a wooden stairs case to complete our custom formalities. I had never experienced such a queue before as I had not seen so many people before. It was quite an experience for me. I was 11 years old then.

We did go on to Melbourne as my mother's cousin had sponsored us to come to Australia. Her house was a reasonably small place; but she managed to put her own two young children in their bedroom with them and she gave us two bedrooms until we got our own accommodation. One room was for my parents and the other for my middle brother and me. I don't really know how long we stayed there because we were so crowded. Soon after we arrived in Australia and we were staying in North Melbourne, I was excitedly going into the city on a tram. I do vividly remember an incident on that Melbourne tram: We spoke Italian at home so my parents asked me a question in Italian so I naturally replied in Italian. I was taken aback when a lady - I am being charitable calling her a lady- yelled at me, "Speak bloody English." Today she could be up for discrimination. It is so good to hear so many languages spoken in Brisbane today. On a recent trip to Melbourne we did go on a tram to reminisce, and did hear many languages spoken on that tram. Australia has grown a lot, we no longer have the 'White Australia Policy' instead we now have Multiculturalism. (Sometimes I wonder if it will work out).

We recently visited the port of Fremantle on a round Australia cruise. We arrived at Freemantle at 7 am. I could not remember the old wooden structure on the dock. That may have been because we were docked at a different place or things were so different after some fifty years. . My wife and I recently went on an organized tour of Egypt, I recently saw a patient that lived in Embramia,

Alexandria, Egypt. He went to the same school as I did back then. He was in my older brother's class. He never fails to remind me that at 4 years old; I used to hate going to school. He also tells me that I used to soil my pants on the bus. My brother was so embarrassed that he would change my pants, but I don't know what he did with my soiled underpants. I still see this lovely person socially. Although he is now quite elderly (80); he does have all his faculties about him. This patient wanted me to get him an up to date map of Embramia so he could compare it to what he recollected of the place. I was able to get him a map of the suburbs of Alexandria as they are today; when he saw the map; he tells me that not very much has changed.

When we visited Alexandria we called in to a beach on the Mediterranean Sea there I saw a rock at the edge of the water. When I saw that rocky outcrop memories started to flow back to me; I recalled that my older brother used to take me fishing there. We went on an organized shore tour Albany in Western Australia when we were on another cruise round Australia; we were in a bus travelling up a hill to see a Light Horse barracks museum. My wife became very concerned because she thought I was losing my mind. I kept repeating "It is the monument that is in Port Said, are we in Port Said?" It is the exact same monument that was at the end of a pier in Port Said. The monument was getting damaged during the Suez war so the Australian Army brought it back to Albany where the Light Horse Regiment was formed. When we got right up to the monument; we saw of some of the actual bullet holes that were made in the base of the monument during the Suez war. During our recent trip to Egypt, we found out the reason for this skirmish. Apparently President Nasser wanted money from the USA to build the upper Aswan dam but the USA kept on putting him off as they were friends with Britain, he has already crossed swords with Britain so he ended up taking full control of the Suez Canal. President Nasser lacked the technology to build the Aswan dam so he invited the Russians to help him. The cold war was still on, so of course the Russians were only too happy to help. Before the dam was filled, a joint task force of several nations painstakingly dismantled a historic tomb of a Pharaoh and reconstructed it on higher ground. Interestingly, they had to build reinforcing behind the reconstructed tomb; whereas the original structure did not need more reinforcing. Evelyn and I kept on wondering what happened to that very intelligent early Egyptian society when it is compared to today's Egyptian society. They built such things as the pyramids and the sphinxes, they transported stones great distances without modern vehicles, they lifted great weights without the aid of cranes; their paintings and building have lasted 4000 years and they have did not have any of the present tools. The museums are full of their beautiful artefacts. There are private collections also of their beautiful artefacts. We were told so many things by our guide that was studding Egyptian History at the Egyptian University in Cairo. It was not until the historians found a tablet that allowed them to translate hieroglyphics. The stone tablet translated the hieroglyphic to ancient Greek. The historians already knew how to read ancient Greek. The Egyptians had recorded in hieroglyphic how they did things. But before the ancient tablet was found; the historians did not know how to read hieroglyphics. Because of that find they then could read hieroglyphics; so then they found out how the ancient Egyptians built such wonderful things. It was originally believed that slaves built the pyramids but it was then found out that the pyramids were sacred ground so slave were not permitted on those sites. The Nile River used to flood every year (before the Aswan dam was built) so the farmers were unable to work their land. The Pharos gave employment to the farmers during the time that the River Nile flooded. So the pyramids were actually built by farmers and not slaves as was first believed. Incidentally the Nile River the only is river in the world that flows from South to North.

We were truly amazed at the temples. The temples were built in such a way that the day light entered the building no matter what time of the day it was. Another feature of temples that was even more important in the hot Egyptian climate was that the food may have been offered during the day has to be kept cool until the high priests could consume it in the evenings. That room that the offerings were kept in the temple was kept cool by circulating water between the walls of that room. It acted as a 'cool room' to keep the offerings cool until the evening. When you compare these marvellous achievements of that ancient generation with the present generation in the same country you have to ask "where have the past generation gone?" . We visited Cairo Museum and saw Tutankhamen treasures and coffins; they are pleural because he had three coffins. The riches that were buried with him were unbelievable. Using today's DNA technologies they found that young Pharos Tutankhamen died of Malaria; they did find the DNA of the Malaria parasites; so many centuries later; in his remains.

An interesting fact is that a British Archeologist (I think his name is/was Carter) had been looking for Tutankhamen tomb for several years; a grave robber had told him of the gold and the riches that were in the in the tomb. He searched for years but he been unable to find that tomb; eventually his backers telegrammed him from England that they had had enough; they would not send him any more money to continue his search. So he started to pull up his camp; while he was pulling up his tent he noticed that the sand kept on falling down a tent peg hole; that he had just pulled up; so he realize that he had pitched his tent right over the tomb he was looking for. The tombs in the Valley of the Kings were another wonder. The ancient catacombs in Alexandria were amazing; they were dug into the desert sand and were many floors deep. There were so many wonderful relics I do hope that they are well preserved. Unfortunately the ancient paintings and the temples are not always carefully respected as visitors flock to these sites. Some people unknowingly rest or rub their rug sack on the pillars and other artefacts.

The new Alexandria library is phenomenal; one can access their web site and thereby have access to 7 floors of their reference books. It was built by a consortium of nation.

CHAPTER TWO

———— ◆))·((————

W hen we recently went to Melbourne to visit my parents; that were still there at that time; we laughed when we took our children and their friends to see the Victoria Market. The children and their friends sat on a wall and played a game that they called "Spot the Aussie". The Market has many Asian traders now selling all manner of goods. Many years ago, there were a lot of Jewish traders; that dealt with many beautiful materials. Some were excellent tailors as well. In fact; when I was still a student in Melbourne; one tailors from Melbourne markets made me a pair of tailor made trousers. I do miss those days. Everyone remembers and says that the good old days were so good; but is it just that we remember them? Some of the changes that have occurred since are much better than the in good old days; for just for examples; the changes to the discrimination laws and the great food menus that are now available. Many migrants, from the many varied cultures, can have a welcoming attitude and be many can also be so generous that it is so delightful that it enrich our wonderful country.

Most of us do appreciate the good changes that the many different cultures have brought to this country; however there are still some unkind individuals that make discriminating comments; luckily though, they are in the minority! So, after we arrived in Melbourne we stayed with our sponsors a while, until my parents were able to rent two rooms in Pascoe Vale. Australia was quite under developed so accommodation was not easy to get (it was 1953). In those days it was difficult and too expensive to rent a whole house. Whilst I was there I attended a Catholic primary school run by an order of nuns. I believed I spoke English well as I had attended a British Boys school in Egypt. When I first started to school, I was repeatedly told to speak "bloody English". It does shows how attitudes have changed so that even children used to decimate then; today it would be very different.

My step father worked very hard. As well as having a full time factory job, he remembered from his youth that he has been taught how repair shoes so he started to do so and he also joined a band to play at some gig on some evenings; remember he was a professional musician; he did My parents eventually bought a low set single fronted house in North Melbourne.

My parents then took me to the local Christian Brothers secondary School in North Melbourne and enrolled me there. They were able to negotiate reduced fees; I think it was because we were migrants. I did my secondary school there (at the Christian Brothers School in North Melbourne). I am grateful to the Brothers as they took me on with reduced fees. I am still very grateful for their generosity.

While I was at that school; several very humorous incidences happened there; although I did not think so at the time. The first happened in fourth or fifth grade. In those days physical punishment was acceptable. I had misbehaved; I don't recall what I did but it must have been punishable by the strap. The teacher gave me a choice; you can have the strap on your palm of your hand or on your back side. I chose my backside as I thought I would be clever. Before I went to get the strap on my backside I quickly slid an exercise book under my shorts of my school uniform. The sound that the strap made when the strap hit the exercise book alerted the teacher of my "trick". He made me remove the exercise book and then flogged me twice as hard.

In the senior years I used to ride my bike to school; on the way to school there was a very steep hill with a terribly cold head wind; this wind was especially cold in Melbourne winters. On one very cold winter's day I decided that I would put my long trousers uniform on top of my pyjamas to ride my bike to school. That morning when I got to school, the school nurse was there to examine us. You can just imagine my embarrassment when I had to undress! I did not feel so bad because some other pupils had done the same.

At one time; I remember the whole class that was made up of 45 pupils, including the teacher; had spent the better part of a whole period trying unsuccessfully to solve a mathematical problem. The head master was the our math's, science and chemistry teacher offered to give any child that would solve the problem a chocolate bar. I spent a lot of time that night to solve that problem; in the end it was reasonably simple. The next morning the headmaster asked if anyone has a solution to the problem. I very proudly replied that I had the solution to the problem. He, unbelieving said, "Show me on the black board". At that time the teacher did use chalk and a black board and chalk to rite on the black board. As I walk up to the board to demonstrate to the teacher and the whole class the solution to the elusive problem my chest was all the way out. I did show how the problem was easily solved. He then had to acknowledge that I did have the right solution to the elusive problem, He then took me to the tuck shop to get me the promised chocolate bar; going to the tuck with him was a much greater buzz than getting the chocolate bar.

I do some have bad memories too of certain bad punishments. I was often a few minutes late, so I had to wait outside the class until the teacher was ready to punish my action. The punishment was to be six of "the best as the best" as he used to call six straps on the out stretched palm. As I was late again the punishment grew to "six of the best" on each hand. To boot it all, he was a very big man. He would swing the strap behind his back to get a full swing on the strap as he would give you" six of the best". Mind you I was not the only one to experience this punishment. After the strapping I would be allowed to go to my place in the class. I would often sit on my hands in an attempt to quell the pain. I would do so especially in the cold Melbourne winters. The teacher would then walk down the aisle to my desk and ask me "why it was it that I was not working?" I would then attempt to get my numb hands from under my backside; and start working; he would then hit me across the knuckles with the edge of a steel ruler. Luckily my hand were still numb so it did not hurt that much. Years later, after many years after that we had left school and I had graduated as a doctor I did come across him again. I will later talk of another past pupil that refused to come to dinner with him.

Our headmaster had teaching as well as the administration duties. He happened to be teaching us when he was called to the office. He gave us permission to talk, as long as we were discussing our work, while he was away from the class. I was discussing a mathematical problem with my desk mate; so as the noise in the classroom got louder and louder so did my voice got louder and louder! Incidentally my desk mate was an especially large person you could say he was fat; he used to eat two meat pies for morning tea; he did die of a heart attack when he was only forty three; rest his soul. . I was so engaged in our math's discussion that I did not realize the headmaster had returned to the classroom; although the rest of the class was suddenly silent my partner and I were still talking loudly, He heard my voice, so he called out to me, "Garsia if that is your attitude pick up your books and go". I did not hear the first part of his statement "if that is your attitude" but all I heard was "pick up your books and go". He again said "Well!" I looked at him in amazement; after all I had been discussing mathematical problems with my desk partner as he had requested. He again repeated, "Well!" So what was I to do? He had directed me to do go, so I picked up my books and left. I did not realize at the time, why he looked so surprised; after all he has told me to go.

When I went to school the next day, I found out I had been expelled! Imagine the panic? At that time in Victoria we did external examinations and I could not sit for my examination unless the school verified that I had completed grade 12. It was only 2 weeks before I could sit for my final year but I was expelled before I had finished. My parents' even though they were so busy; made the effort came with me to the school. They pleaded with the headmaster to let me finish grade 12; even though they explained that it was all a big miss understanding; he was adamant that would not have me back. They again tried to explain why and how the miss understanding happened he still refused to have me back. He just would not listen to their explanation. Finally he agreed to certify that I completed grade 12 but he still refused to take me back to finish my school year. As it turned out, the expulsion was the best thing that happened to me. Before the final examinations; during those two weeks, I worked and swatted very hard. As a result I managed to get several 2nd class honours; that was enough to get me an interview with the Dean of the Medical Faculty at the University of Melbourne; the interview enabled me to be admitted to the Medical course and the rest they say "is history".

CHAPTER THREE

———————◆))◦◦((◆———————

During my medical course some things happened that are worth reporting. Medical students always have been known to get up to funny pranks. The first one that I vividly remember happened when we started University. The initiation prank involved the freshmen; as we were called then; we were to go to the centre of the city and urinate on the left back wheel of a car; of course it was to be in full view of the public and to make sure that a policeman could see us. A senior student had found there was a law that it was still legal to urinate on the left back wheel of a vehicle. Apparently the police could not do anything about it. Although urinating in public was illegal.

On my second year we started dissecting; for our anatomy lessons. The whole morning was taken up by these lessons. On the first day in the dissecting room; my mother gave me corned beef sandwiches for my lunch. The body that the University supplied for my anatomy lessons was that of an old derelict that had died and had been in water for some time. His flesh was like corned beef. Needless to say, after the morning in the anatomy room, I could not face my lunch. I do eat most things but I still cannot stomach corn beef.

During the second year we started anatomy lessons that involved dissection of cadavers; I recall an anatomy student stealing body parts from the dissecting room and putting them in his pocket. When he got on a tram he asked the conductor if he wanted a hand; the conductor replies that would be good as the tram was very crowded. He produced from his pocket the real thing -a real hand that he had stolen from the anatomy room! Everybody on the tram was disgusted and flabbergasted. That student got into a lot of trouble the next day at the University.

My Medical course went over for six years. The first year comprise of lectures in biology, chemistry, physics and an unrelated subject; in order to ensure that we were not too narrow in our course. The second year was more medical with lecture in anatomy, histology and biochemistry. In our third year we did learn about the medical conditions. At the end of the 3rd. year and at the beginning of 4th year we started our clinical training. We started at the teaching hospitals, the Royal Melbourne Hospital and St Vincent's Hospital.

I started at St Vincent's Hospital. I was very eager to see a delicate operation. So I looked up the theater list for that day; there was an eye operation, using a microscope, scheduled for that morning. I thought that was for me; I rushed to the 4th floor where the operating theatres were. I quickly changed into theatre clothing and proceeded to theatre 4. However I got mixed up because of my sense of direction (of right and left); I turned right instead of left. I ended up in theatre 3. In that theatre there was a hip repair; so I was confronted with a large 6ft+ orthopaedic surgeon and frail little women on an orthopaedic bed. The patient was strapped up with her legs in stirrups. He was hammering the new head of the femur into her femur. With every hammer blow the poor old lady shook all over. It was far from delicate so; that was my introduction to delicate surgery. I quickly realized that I was in the wrong theatre so I left and went into the correct theatre, there I did see the delicate (eye) surgery. In the hospital casualty, Medical students used to get some terrible jobs. I will never forget one of these jobs. I was on duty one evening when an old man came in. He had not washed for several weeks and he was very constipated so he had not moved his bowels for over a week. He had deep leg ulcers so much so that the proud flesh had grown through his long johns. I got the job to slowly cut away his long johns so that his sores could be dressed; I then had to manually disinpact his constipated bowel. The smell was so terrible and it took a long time to do the job properly, I often had to stop for a while in order to compose myself to go on.

On another occasion, I remember that several student doctors were in one of the cubicles in casualty. We all were very sympathetic to this young mother. She had come in with her 2+ year unconscious boy child with a skull fracture. The history was that the toddler had fallen out his cot. When the registrar came into the cubicle, he immediately directed us to call the police. We were all amazed. We eventuated found out that he had conferred with his the honorary (as they were called then). I presumed that he told the registrar that the child's fracture was not consistent with a fall from his cot. When the police came and interview the woman; it turned out that the women was having a loud argument with her Defacto partner; the toddler tried to intervene by getting between them. The Defacto step father picked up the child and heaved him against the wall; it was in this way that the child got this terrible skull fracture. Incidentally the child never regained consciousness and died.

The lesson we all learnt was to be always aware that the history we obtained is consistent with the presenting injury, and if we are unsure always involve an expert that are better suited to detective work. We are not policemen so it is very difficult to know when to disbelieve our patient.

Back in 1964, during my time at the teaching hospital, I learned another very interesting and fascinating thing. How technology has progressed in every aspect of science. Some of the specialists were experimenting with a machine using sound to map muscles etc. At the time we did not know that that machine would become the modern ultrasound machine of today. They have become common place, and in some cases they are a preferable as the investigation tool of choice. Another incident that happened back then; a technology professor would now probably turn in his grave if he found out how computers have taken over our world. He took us to show us the early computers; we all had to wear masks and gowns when we entered this air conditioned and dust free room. It was full of large reel to reel tape recorders. He told us that all this fancy and expensive equipment could do was sort out addresses. He then proceeded to show us another room that had a punch card system; he told us mark my word this is the future. I think punch card systems would only be found in museums now.

Open heart surgery was unknown, as the bypass machine has not yet been developed. So the early heart operations required the patient to go into an ice bath so that their metabolism was so slowed that surgeon could get time to operate on the heart. My middle brother had open heart surgery by the time that the bypass machine had been developed; he was in intensive care for four weeks. Medical advances have gone a long way since; my older brother also had a quadruple bypass recently and he was out of intensive care the next day, walking the following day and home in four days. I am totally fascinated when I go into a hospital now to see the progress that has occurred since my student days. Is it any wonder that we are required to upgrade our knowledge by personal development programs?

CHAPTER FOUR

I got a Victorian State Government scholarship. That scholarship did not pay a living allowance so I did many and various jobs. These jobs included working for a taxi company to cleaning their filthy toilets. It was during this job of cleaning toilets that when I stood on an old toilet pan to reach up high to remove some spider webs the pan collapsed and I fell into the bowl. Another time I used dilute caustic soda to try and remove old urine stains, lovely is it not! Another job I did was to complete surveys door to door. It paid well however because they were infrequent, they were not enough to pay the bills; so I tried selling or tutoring but I was not cut out to be a sales man or a tutor. Hospitality in the hotel industry offered me many opportunities to earn extra dollars. I worked as a bar man; but my main job was waiting on tables. There are many experiences that I recall, however I will only talk about some of the ones that stand out in my memories. When I was a waiter at a five star hotel, we were serving supper when a well-known T.V. host came in with his guests and colleagues. A fellow waiter was serving their coffee and he asked how they would like their coffee? The T.V. host smugly replied to that the waiter "I like my coffee like I like my women; strong and sweet", without any hesitation the waiter replied yes sir "black or white". I do wish that I could be so spontaneous as he was.

The hotel I was working at, had water fall as a feature in the foyer. I was a drink waiter at that time; one very busy Saturday evening;

a very inebriated patron asked me where the male toilet was. I was coming from the bar with a heavy tray with many drinks; I replied that "it was just past the waterfall" but because I did heavy tray with many drinks I did not take him there. He must not have heard me properly, because on my way back to the bar I saw this man urinating in the waterfall. The hotel manager saw as he was urinating in the waterfall so naturally he was very cross with him; he went and chastised him loudly. This man waited outside till the end of the night; as we all left the hotel about 1am; he punched the poor manager on the chin very hard. I felt guilty because it did seem that it was partly my fault because I did not actually take him to the toilet.

At another venue, on another evening, the barman asked me if I could drive him home, I said "sure!" then I asked "where do you want to go?" With a great smirk on his face he said "I will go anywhere you would like to take me!" I had learnt a saying that seemed very appropriate at times like these. The statement is "Backs against the wall." It did relate to picking up the soap that fell on to the floor in the shower but that saying seemed very appropriate in this case.

On another occasion my mates and I worked as kitchen hands at the cadet camp as cooks' assistants. A lot of the cadets under officer were very arrogant and down putting to us, so we decided to teach them a lesson. We prepared the tomato soup for their formal dinner. First we got some Epsom salts from the stores (their medical center) and then we put these aperients into the tomato soup. Apparently the soup was very nice because many of the cadets and under officers had second servings. Before the next course was served there was a long queue to the latrines. The under officers must have realized what we had done because they were then very respectful to us from then on.

I often worked with a Jewish Kosher caterer. I was seen as one of them because of my long nose in fact the caterer often called me Ajax at these functions. At one very big reception he needed as many waiters as he could get. He employed a Norwegian sailor; I will call him Fred for the purpose of this discourse. He would get extra work when his ship was in port being repaired and in dry dock. I think it is called moonlighting. On that occasion the reception was for a very traditional Jewish wedding. The men were seated on one side of the hall and the women were on the other side of the hall. The men were separated from the women by a row of plants. The rabbi's sat at the head table with the bride and groom. They started to pray; giving thanks for their meal. In anticipation, the caterer served up the greasy consommé soup as the first course He told us the waiters to wait until the rabbis' had finished their prayers before we served this soup to the guests. Obviously the head table would be first to be served when the rabbis has finished praying.

Fred the sailor, who was again quite inebriated; did not want wait until the rabbis had finished praying; he took the soup to the head table and started to serve the soup but the rabbis. Had not finished praying; as the rabbis chanted in prayer they were bowing up and down. Fred waited for his opportunity; as the main rabbi's head was upright he quickly put the soup bowl under the rabbi's head. Picture now; as the rabbi continued praying his beard kept going into the greasy soup; His long grey beard was dripping with the greasy soup as he kept on praying chanting and bowing up and down. The rabbi continued to pray for several minutes so this hilarious sight continued for some time. I guess it was funny to watch but not for the rabbi. Naturally Fred never ever again worked with that caterer..

At one time I got a job working on a cruise ship. In order to re-enter Australia I needed a passport quickly. At that time it was quicker to be naturalized to get the reentry visa than to wait for a passport. I recall all I has to do was swear allegiance to Australia in order to be naturalized so I went to the Melbourne's Lord Mayor to get my naturalization certificate. With my naturalization certificate I was able to go onto the cruise ship and return to Australia. The job did not start till we got to Sydney but we boarded the ship in Melbourne, so we had several days before we started to work.

There were many people that congregated in a small cabin to explore a séance. I was very interested to see what happens at a séance as I had never been to one. Just imagine being crowded in a very small cabin; the mediums voice was the only one that could be heard. She was calling on a spirit by using her Ouija Board. Suddenly Fred; yes it was the same Fred that I had spoken about previously was also on board; burst through the door wanting to know where the spirit was. He meant where this spirit, the alcohol was. Needless to say that was the end of the séance.

I had an old (1951) Vauxhall Velox during the earlier years of my medical course. The Vauxhall's gearbox was always breaking down. The synchromesh ring would not allow me to go into 3rd gear so I would have to drive in 2nd gear. It did it so often that I could take the gearbox out on the side of the road; fix it and then put it back in the car in about an hour. After working late on one evening at a waiting job; I was driving home when the gearbox of the Velox played up again. I could not be bothered fixing the gearbox that night; as I could drive the car in 2nd gear as long as I would not stop. As I could not stop I did go through an orange light; as I went across the lights a car hit me very slightly. I drove on slowly. It was very funny to see driver of the car that collided with me running beside my car, to apologize for hitting me.

On another occasion, late at night again; the gear box broke down. I was driving home in 2nd gear but I had to stop at a red light so the car stalled and then the motor stopped. I can clearly remember that it was at the Kew junction. When I tried to start it again it would not start because it was still in 2nd gear.. A huge truck behind me started toting me. He did not realize I was stalled and I could not start the car. He stepped out of his truck and started abusing me very angrily. I was frightened by the truck driver as he was so angry and he did not want to listen to any of my explanations; just then a Fiat Toppolino (they were tiny cars) pulled up and he also got of his car. He was so large that he had taken the front seat of the car and drove the car sitting on the back seat. He did realize that my car was stalled and I was having trouble starting it. He told the very irate truck driver in no uncertain words to stop abusing me and to get back in his fucking truck and drive around me. I was so relieved when the second driver intervened.

CHAPTER FIVE

———————————————— ◀))) · ((▶ ————————————————

During the second year of my medical course in 1962 I had a car accident in my 1951 Vauxhall Velox. I was travelling along Sydney road, one of the main roads in Melbourne. I came to an intersection controlled by traffic lights. The traffic lights had just turned orange as I got to the intersection, so I proceeded (as you do). Stopping suddenly could cause an accident as another car was following closely behind me almost tail gating me.

A car stopped that was the lights on the other side of the intersection, (remember the lights were still red for him) took off right away believing that the lights has turned green for him, so he collided with me in the middle of the intersection. At that time, many eye witnesses were prepared to testify as to what happened; however (at the time) I did not think that I had sustained any injury or that there was any damage to either car so I did not take any eye witnesses names and addresses. Apart from the eye being blood shot because I had hit my left eye on the steering wheel I could see perfectly well so I thought that there was no physical damage. There did not seem to be any damage to the cars either. Month later; I started finding that I was getting blind spots in the left eye; it was then that I was I diagnosed that I had developed a retinal detachment due to the car accident at the Royal Melbourne Eye and Ear Hospital. I then contacted the driver of the other car but he denied everything that had really happened. Always do take eye witnesses names as you do not know what can happen latter. I was admitted right away to the hospital. A truly lovely Ophthalmologist repaired my retinal detachment. At that time I was restricted to bed for four weeks. I was not allowed to strain in any way! Just imagine how difficult it was to pass a bowel motion into a bed pan without straining. At my eye operation I apparently did do funny things during the anaesthetic; that and caused them some concern. When I got back to the ward I discovered that my upper right incisor was very loose. The nurses gave me several versions of what has happened. One such story was that my heart had stopped during the operation and that the anaesthetist had to incubate me in a hurry; so it was in this way that they damaged my one of prominent upper incisor teeth. That explanation sounded feasible. I guess I will never know what really happened as I was not told by any doctor that was at my operation. I could not leave my tooth alone as I like to fiddle with the loose tooth, so my prominent incisor tooth eventually came out. I eventually got a dental plate, however I hated wearing it. I was so happy when my wife gave away my suit with my false tooth in the suit pocket.

Getting back to my sight, after the repair of the retinal detachment I did attend for a specialist review. At the specialists review; I had lost much of sight in that left eye. I had developed a central venous thrombosis (a clot) and the detachment had reoccurred. The Ophthalmologist readmitted me immediately to hospital again; it meant another 4 weeks on my back. During that stay in hospital my second brother got married. It was a great thrill as he and his new wife, still in their formal wedding clothes, came to visit me in the hospital.

The insurance payout for my eye injury only covered my medical expenses. The ophthalmic surgeon very kindly agreed to waive his fees.

With the money that the specialist let me keep I bought a second hand white Volkswagen and I later sold the Vauxhall Velox. The white Volkswagen was my pride and joy.

CHAPTER SIX

I was at the Royal Woman's' Hospital in Melbourne, during my 5th year of the medical course while I did the rotation to learn about women's health. Evelyn, my future wife as it turned out, was doing her post graduate certificate in midwifery at the same hospital. There were two redheads at the hospital that I fancied; I was very attracted to redheads. I thought my wife had to be was a natural redhead as she originates from Scotland; her complexion was pale and consistent with red heads. I did accuse the other girl of dying her hair red; she was really a red head. Evelyn really has brown hair and did dye her hair. I had a twenty cent bet with another student, he was also interested in Evelyn. The bet was that I could get her to come out with me. He accepted the bet but he countered with another twenty cents bet, that he would get her to go out with him. We both got her to go out with us. As she did go out with both of us nobody won the bet.

On Friday nights the hospital food was yucky; it was some terribly cooked fish; so she welcomed and accepted the invitation from him to take her to tea. She chose to go out for dinner with him before she returned to duty. I asked her if I could take her home, as it was her weekend off she agreed. But I did not find out where she lived before I asked her to drive her home. I still had the Vauxhall as I had not yet got the Volkswagen; she lived in a suburb called Forrest Hills which was on the other side of town from where I lived. Luckily my car did not break down that night.

As I drove into Evelyn's street I knew I was done for. It was called Husband road. I really was head over heels about her already, but I told her it was the street name that did it. Incidentally, the other student is now is a Professor of Obstetrics and Gynaecology in New Zealand

Soon after I got my white Volkswagen; because Evelyn had to attend lectures for her course in her own time at another hospital; I let Evelyn borrow my white Volkswagen car. I did anxiously meet her on her return from the lecture; it was really to check on my pride and joy. Evelyn had given her friends a lift back from the lecture; to my surprise and amazement; I watched as one girl after another piled out of the car. How on earth did she get 10 girls in a Volkswagen Beetle? She had them sitting on each other knees; she even had got some girls in the narrow luggage compartment at the back of the Volkswagen. Of course that was before seat belts became compulsory. I bragged about having 10 girls in my car from that day on. At that time students had to attend to twenty deliveries, the trainee midwives also had to get twenty deliveries record in their practice books in order to graduate. So there was a competition to get the required numbers of deliveries between the midwives and the medical students. The trainee nurses would call the students to late to attend to the deliveries; so by the time that the student got to the labour ward from our quarters it was too late. So the student worked a roster system; A student would stay in the labour ward and alert the next student of an impending delivery- in time.

During that time all the medical students wore all white shirts, white trousers, white shoes, white belts and white bow ties. I don't remember if we had to wear white underpants too! Any way Evelyn was on night duty. after having been at the beach all day. She had a ward full of screaming Italian ladies. A student, of very similar appearance to me, appeared behind her; he said to her "you should learn to speak Italian so that you can do better with the patients". He then he left. At that time there were many Italians in Melbourne. It was my turn to be in the ward but I had no idea of what had gone on before. So when I heard so many ladies were yelling. I told her "to speak slower to the ladies" so that they could understand her. Evelyn does have a slight a accent; she replied "if you are so bloody smart do it yourself" and threw the bed pans at me and stormed off; I thought that she was so cranky and irritable because she has been at the beach all day and did not like having to wear stiffly starched uniforms. Apparently she waited in the pan room until she calmed down. I do speak Italian; I settle the ladies down and I took their observations like their BPs, pulses and urine samples. I tested their urine and I wrote them all down for her. When she came back she had to eat humble pie; she really apologized when she realized I had made the ladies settle and taken and written all their observations for her. She also realized that it was not me that has made the previous statements to her; that was really why she had been so upset.

During the fifth year of the medical course at Melbourne University the medical students were required to do a country experience. I did choose to do my two weeks with a country general practice in the town of Warburton. The practice I chose did have access to hospital beds at the local country hospital. At that time general practitioner's did have access to hospital beds. Anyway, I was in the toilet when I was thinking how much I missed my girlfriend so I decided to write her a love letter. The toilet paper was readily available, so I wrote her the letter on the toilet paper. It must have been a really loving letter, because she kept and treasured the letter for years. It later became a great conversation piece with our friends. During that rotation in my 5th year of my Medical course at Melbourne University, Evelyn and were both at the Royal Woman's' Hospital. My group found out that our Obstetric & Gynaecology professor loved Stilton cheese. My study group asked me to get some Stilton cheese, to have at an afternoon tea with our obstetrics and gynaecology Professor. We did not realize that he would only eat very little off it, as it has such a strong taste. I had bought a quarter of a kilogram of the cheese. So after the afternoon tea with him I took the remainder of the cheese to my room in the student doctors' quarters. It did not only have a strong taste but it stunk. I was still courting Evelyn when she came to visit me at the student quarters. She offered to wash my socks for me as she thought the putrid smell was from my dirty socks. We had a good laugh when I told her it was not my socks and I got her to smell the cheese. I don't remember what I eventually did with the cheese. I probably threw it out.

When I asked Evelyn to marry me, I asked her to meet my parents. She was quite terrified as I had told her about them. They wanted me to marry an Italian girl. Even though we were not Italian somehow we did adopt the Italian label. Evelyn is Scottish and as well as that she was not a Catholic; she was Church of England at that time. The meeting did not go well; they told her about my previous girl friends they brought out to her my previous girl friends' letters trying to put her off. It did not work. We have been happily married nearly 46 years and have 5 lovely children.

One night I took my fiancé, (by that time we were engaged), to the pictures, on the way back to the nursing home I took her parking at Elwood beach. We had taken her green Volkswagen on that occasion;. A very funny thing happened; but at the time it seemed it was very embarrassing but now it does seem very funny! Her green Volkswagen was supposed to be a 1962 model as it had a fuel gauge. However it still had a reserve fuel tank operated by a lever in the lower part of the floor next to the cars' pedals. The reserve tank was there in the earlier models before the fuel gauges became standard equipment. It was there to remind the driver that he needed more fuel if he had to use the reserve tank. But I was not aware that there were models with both the reserve tank that had the levers near the floor and the pedals of the car as well as the fuel gauge. We had finished parking so we started to go back to the nursing home but the car would not start no matter what we tried. Finally I called the R.A.C.V. the service man came out within the hour. With a big smirk on his face he told us he knew what we were doing, with that he just lent down at the front of the driver's side of the car and turned the lever for the reserve petrol tank. When the lever is accidentally placed in the upright position all the petrol to the motor is turned off. He proceeded to tell us that it often happened and it was a common occurrence with that particular model of car. After he turned the lever I did immediately start the car. Can you just imagine how embarrassed we were at the time?

CHAPTER SEVEN

Before we got married matters were made worse because of the family disagreement. They started as soon as we stated to discuss our plans for marriage. Even though it is for the couple to work out as it is their day, my parents wanted me to get married in our parish. Evelyn's parents said it was the bride's parents' decision and they wanted us to get married closer to them. However they were good about it and they did not pressure us. Remember that she lived on the other side of Melbourne! I think you know exactly what it is like at that time before a marriage, one side pulling one way' wanting their way the other side pulling the other way and wanting their way. The emotions were running high! We finally did manage to reach a compromised to every body's satisfaction. We chose a church half way. We chose a church in East Melbourne, Evelyn believed it would be better for the children if she became Catholic. Anyway, the high Church of England is not so far removed in its beliefs from the Catholic religion. A lovely priest from St Francis Church in Melbourne took Evelyn through the lessons to become a Catholic. We wanted that priest from St Francis to be the celebrant for the wedding. The wedding was to take place in East Melbourne. It was another parish church, so another parish priest. Luckily there was a football cup final on the day that we wanted to get married so the parish priest at East Melbourne was very happy to let us use his church and our priest so that he could go to the match. Traditionally, the bride cannot be early for her wedding. So the wedding cars drove round and around the block, before they drove into the church. I did think all sought of thoughts whiles she was being fashionably late. Did she change her mind? Had she had an accident on the way to the church? What had happened? I was so relieved to see her when she finally arrived. I do tease her, that she is still following that principle of being late for appointments, but then again she did have five children to get ready. The priest that just married humorously told us; while we were signing the marriage register; not to consummate the marriage in case he has not married us correctly; after all he did not have much practice marring couples and could not guarantee that everything had been done right. Off course he was just joking but it took us back a first.

We had the reception at Evelyn's parents place. Her younger brother one her brothers Aian who was only sixteen at the time ended up being very drunk on Slivovitch (Hungarian Brandy.) by the end of the evening; At the end of the wedding reception we got ready to go to our honeymoon in Surfers Paradise. Before we were married we used each have a Volkswagen. My Volkswagen was white and hers was green, incidentally before we were married we used to race each other along Burwood road. We did take hers (the green one) on our honeymoon because her father had just serviced it. After many good byes, we got into her car to drive off; as I tried to drive off it the car would not go anywhere. It would only rev. Her father reassured me that the car was o.k. so I got out of the car to see what was wrong with the car. There was nothing wrong with the car; her older brothers had lifted the car onto blocks, so the car wheels were off the ground. That was why the car would not go anywhere. After lots of laughter her brothers lifted the car off the blocks and we were away. They had tied a lot of empty cans to the back of the car so when we drove off we made a lot of noise. I stopped a few meters from the house to untie the cans. They had written all over the car just married. However they had used shaving cream, not knowing that it was terrible for car's paint, so I did wipe it all off.

We had not booked a place thinking it was August and places would not be too busy, and anyway I did not know how far we would get before we wanted to stop. On the way the accelerator cable hole had not been plugged so the cold air kept coming up my leg. It did not seem to matter as to how I placed my leg to avoid the freezing cold draught as a drove; that it made any difference. So I put on my pyjamas to cover my good clothes and got under the car to plug the offending hole. By the way, I only wear pyjamas in hospital. It was now almost 11pm when we arrived at a town called Euroa. The town was as busy, like Burke Street in Melbourne on a Saturday morning. I asked the locals why it was so busy. They told me that they were having a motor cycle race meeting. In any case there would not be any accommodation in the town, perhaps I could find some accommodation in another town close by. They gave me directions to the hotel (pub) in that town, so I went off to find this hotel.

When I got to the place, I rang the doorbell several times. A large seedy man finally answered the doorbell, He greeted me with, "Yerr, what do you want?" I realized it was not a place I wanted to be at and so I quickly said that I was the wrong place and left. Deciding to go on and try the next town, we drove on into the night. We got to the next town at 12 midnight. The town is called Benalla.

Again the town was very busy, like Burke Street in Melbourne is on a Saturday morning. I asked again asked one of the local why was the town so busy? He replied, "We are having a ploughing festival the whole of weekend". So again no accommodation! What a good start to our honeymoon! So again we went on. I was feeling terrible that I had not made arrangements for the accommodation for our honeymoon before our wedding. Just before we got to the next town we spotted a motel displaying a vacancy sign. I quickly pulled into their driveway and went to reception area. It was now close to 1am and we were very tired. I rang the after hour's bell. A lovely lady came to attend to us. She immediately recognized that we were newlyweds. I am sure that it was not difficult to recognize that we were newlyweds so; she told us she was very sorry but she only had one room available and it only had a three quarter bed. We really did not care as we were so tired and besides a three quarter bed would do us just fine. The room was not very big so the bed was against the wall. Being a gentleman I naturally took the inside position. In the morning I woke up finding myself pinned against the wall. After all we had just got married so I really did not mind as we had just got married and I loved Evelyn being very close to me.

In the morning the fun really started! When I went for a shower; there was only cold, very cold water. I quickly showered and I went back to my room shivering, only wearing my towel around my waist. When I started to get dressed with my clean clothes, confetti went everywhere. My brother had patiently put confetti between each layer of clothing in my suitcase. When I tried to put on my socks they too were filled with confetti. I had to empty them first. There where confetti all over the room. Evelyn had a very similar time with her shower and putting on fresh clothes. Tiding the room confetti was quite a task.

When we went to front desk, to check out the same lovely lady receptionist from the night before (or the early morning that day) apologized to us because there was no hot water. She explained that some naughty children had run the hot water taps till there was none left. Their parents discovered their mischief too late. Children will be children everywhere! The rest of the trip was uneventful.

After checking out we drove on to Surfers Paradise. We stayed at the old Pink Panther motel. A fellow medical student had arranged for us to stay with his grandparents. They were the owner-operators the Pink Panther motel. It has since been replaced by a large resort style motel of the same name. They were lovely people. They suggested it might be nice for us to experience another location as well as Surfers Paradise. They did own a duplex at Brunswick Heads. They asked us if we would like to go there as well. I had not completed my degree, so I was worried about the coming years so we were on a tight budget. They must have red my expression so they explained that we could have the duplex for a few days rent free; we then did jump at the chance.

We first celebrated our honeymoon in Surfers Paradise. We went for a special honeymoon dinner at the Chevron Hotel restaurant. That hotel has been replaced by a large residential complex of the same name. I previously stated that I had been a waiter during my student days in order to financially support myself, I had been a waiter at the hotel of the same name in Melbourne. At the Chevron Hotel restaurant on the Gold Coast I met many waiters I had previously worked with. We had ordered Crepes Suzette for our deserts; so the waiter was to cook the crepes at the table. So when it came to cooking our deserts, the waiters were extremely generous with the liqueurs, (they kept on pouring more and more). I tease Evelyn that I married her because she is such a cheap drunk, but then again so am I.

So after wine with our dinner, then the creeps we were quite drunk. We went for a walk to try to sober up after our dinner. Somehow we found ourselves on the roof of the hotel. The hotel was undergoing renovation and extensions. There were no barriers on the roof, as they did not expect any lay persons on the roof. Evelyn had to stop me from walking off the top of the building. After that incident we somehow found our way off the roof of the building. We then went window shopping. While we were looking in a shop window my wife tried to walk through the glass window of that shop

The next afternoon we headed for Brunswick Heads. It was afternoon because we had been so pissed the night before that we did only get up until very late. We got to Brunswick Heads late at night. Most residents were in bed so I could not find anybody to ask directions. After a lot of searching; we finally found the place we were looking for. As we opened the front door we were unsure that we were in the right place. The place was beautifully furnished, complete with a crystal cabinet full of crystal glasses and ornaments. In any case we could not ask anybody so we decided to stay there that night. The next morning we checked if in fact we had got the correct unit. We did in fact have to the right unit. They had generously offered their very own beautiful unit for us to stay in. We had a wonderful time in Brunswick Heads.

Brunswick Heads has a wonderful harbour, so we hired a row boat for the afternoon to explore the harbour. The harbour has many dolphins and a lot of wildlife. It was really very funny to see Evelyn so scared when she saw fins swimming near the boat! She though they were sharks. She did not know that they were playful dolphins that were just following us playfully. She was very relieved to find out the fins belonged to friendly playful dolphins. Even to this day it has made a very good story to repeat when I want to tease her.

CHAPTER EIGHT

s I was still a University student in final year of my course when we got married and I had yet to graduate. I was quite concerned as if our financial situation would see me through till I graduated. If I did not graduate then what would be my options? Evelyn was working, but as it turned out she got pregnant so she would then have to give up work. It was quite a worrying time so we were on a very tight budget; on our return trip to Melbourne we did not stay in a motel but we slept in the car. When it was time to sleep we pulled up into a truck stop. It was so dark that night that I did not see where the truck stop was. We spent the night in the Volkswagen freezing. It did not seem that whatever we used to cover ourselves with kept us warm, so all we did was fight over the covers all night. As well the car was very uncomfortable to sleep in. When the dawn broke we realized that the truck stop was at top of a high mountain; that was why we had been so cold that night. There was a consolation the view were great from the top of that mountain. The rest of the trip was uneventful.

We started to look for reasonable accommodation when we got to Melbourne. I wanted it close to the St Vincent's Hospital and it had to be at a reasonable rental. After many telephone calls we found a share house in North Fitzroy. Back then, it was not the posh suburb that it is now. It suited me well because was close by to where I was doing my hospital training at St Vincent's Hospital; Evelyn started work at Cabrini private hospital so she needed a car. Although we still had the two cars, we wanted to sell one. I could walk to St Vincent's Hospital if I needed too. The share accommodation was partly furnished and came with 'pets'. It consisted of a bedroom that was across a common passage way to the dining room and a kitchen. We especially liked the furry rodents (rats) that came with the house and were always sharing with us.

I bought a pair of second hand chairs from an auction room as my fist acquisition. I paid 2 shillings and six pence for them. We were so pleased with our purchase after all it was better than sitting on tea chests.

After a formal medical student's dinner one a hot summer's night, I came home late and I was still in my dinner suit. The night was very hot, as Melbourne can get in summer. During the dinner they had wine on the table. It was the only drink available so we all drank the wine. At 10pm the caterers brought out cold beer; so everyone was hot and thirsty so we quickly drank lots of cold beer. As a result most of us were quite intoxicated.

Tradition has it, that the senior students are to look after the more junior medical students. So I took two of the junior class students that were going my way. We walked to the tram terminus in Swanston Street and caught a tram. It was such a hot night that the canvas shutters that were used to close one side of the trams exit doors as the tram went one way then on the return journey they were alternatively pulled down; had not been pulled down so both sides of the tram were opened. Anyway, as I tried to hold one student from getting off the tram too early as the other student tried to get off from the other side and so on. Thank goodness the tram conductor saw this pantomime and he did close off one side.

We recently visited Melbourne to reminisce. The trams are so very different. When we got on a tram there was no conductor you either had to have a 'smartcard' or you had to purchase you ticket from a machine. You must have the right change to purchase the fare. We did not have the right change so we could not buy the tickets so we got off as soon as we could.

Returning now to the of my formal dinner night when I got home after finally getting both junior students to their stops, I was quite exhausted and I was quite drunk. It seemed that as soon as I got into the cool night air the fresh air hit me, so did the alcohol. When I got home all I wanted to do was lay on the bed for a while, but that would not do for Evelyn. In spite of my pleading Evelyn insisted that I take off my dinner suit. When I finally got up to take off my dinner suit I suddenly got a terrible feeling of nausea so I had to vomit. I ran to the kitchen sink, by this time I was naked. I pleaded with Evelyn to give me some clothes. Remember that the passageway between the kitchen and the bedroom was a shared passageway. She was still angry with me, I presume for being drunk, so she refused to give me any clothes. How could I get back to the bedroom and hope that the other tenants did not see me? I grabbed a tea towel and put in front of me, and I ran across the passage hopping that the old ladies in the house would not see me. It was so late that they were probably in bed; but I was so pissed at that time that I did not think of that. When I finally got to bed I slept like a baby.

I don't think I am describing the situation correctly because babies often have very disturbed nights; in any case it is a very common saying so perhaps I should say that I slept like a rock.

Not long after we were married, Evelyn was still working at Cabrini Hospital; she was driving her Volkswagen to work in her nurses' uniform, including her large white veil; when another car cut her off. She was on Burwood Road, Ivanhoe at the time; she wound down her car window and yelled out an unsavoury phrase in Italian as she had heard my mother use that phrase often. Ivanhoe was a very up market suburb, with many "well to do" Italians living there. I really don't know if it still is so up market today. Many of the ladies then wore white gloves, lots of jewellery and they talked with plumbs in their mouths; I am assuming it still is so. Immediately the driver of the other car that had cut her off backed off and waved her through. The ladies in the street all shook their heads.

When my wife came home, she wanted to know what the phase meant. I asked and insisted that she should never again say it, even if she had heard my mother use the phase so often. I tried to explain the phase is really very rude although it is often used–it is very rude; I again told her; that even though she had heard my mother use it very often; that she should never use it. She insisted that she wanted to know what the phrase meant. I translated the sentence for her. She had told the man to go and get fucked up the back side.

CHAPTER NINE

I learnt several very valuable lessons during my undergraduate years. I will share with you the first very important lesson that I remember well. While I was at the Melbourne Royal Children's Hospital I learned that I must always listen to a child's mother. We were to follow the development of a child that we had delivered during my rotation at the Melbourne Royal Women's Hospital. I went to the child's home and I examined the child. I was then to present my findings of the case and discuss them with a specialist paediatrician at the Melbourne Royal Children's Hospital.

On my return from visiting the child; I thought I had examined the child thoroughly; I presented this case to my experienced supervising paediatrician. I made the 'mistake' in mentioning in passing that the mother had expressed to me a concern about her child's hearing. As I continued reporting that I had not found any cause for her concerns. I thought that my examination was normal and thorough, that I had especially looked at the child's ear drums and they were perfectly normal. He did not seem interested in my finding but he then just about ate me alive he emotively told me that "you must never ignore a mother concerns". He demanded I go back, and ask the mother the reason for her concerns. I then asked how to examine such a young child's hearing? He told me to stand behind and out of the of the child sight and to make a loud noise; I had to have the child's mother look for a reaction, including a started reaction from the child; remember to make sure that the child could not see my shadow anywhere. I dutifully returned and I asked about her concerns and I again re-examine the child in the way I had been told to do so.

She told me her husband and one the child's uncle, were profoundly deaf because there was a genetic problem in the family of a hearing loss; they both wore hearing aids from an early age. She believed the problem is called 'Otosclerosis'. I re-examined the child in the way the paediatrician has instructed me to do so. I had mother watch for any startled reaction from the baby. But there was no reaction; the child did not react no matter what I did out of his sight. I was rather meek when I returned to the hospital and reported my findings to the specialist.

To my relief, he did not chastise me. I think that he knew what I would find. He just told me to organize an urgent appointment for the child to be seen in the E.N.T. outpatients and to have a formal hearing test. I did make an urgent appointment with the ENT department for this baby and to have a formal hearing test.

When the child attended the hospital for his appointment and he was tested formally he was found to be profoundly deaf. He was fitted with bilateral hearing aids. The specialist and the ENT department people explained that it was of the utmost importance that a child has good hearing from birth for normal speech and language development and for development for their reading skills at school later. Nowadays, a Cochlear implant may be the way to go.

Over the next two years, I continued to follow this child's progress; his development and his speech and language development was normal.

CHAPTER TEN

———————⟩⟩·⟨⟨———————

My being a medical student and learning all the symptoms and signs of the various conditions that we as humans suffer; when I developed diarrhoea alternating with constipation, I thought the worse. Had I developed a bowel cancer? I consulted the medical officer for us students. He examined me and prescribed Methylphenidate (Ritalin). I thought hang on, I am not anxious or depressed. At the time anxiety was often treated with Ritalin. Very often patients and (students are no different) have difficulty accepting a mental diagnosis, as most of us prefer a medical diagnosis. That was my introduction to psychiatric medicine.

The brain is part of our body as much as are the other organs; and cannot be thought of as separate it from the body. A psychiatric problem is no different from a medical (physical) diagnosis. I was still very worried, so I asked to be referred to a general physician that I did have a lot of respect for. When I got to see him, he read my file then he looked at me and quite angrily said "don't you waste my time just go". I left so angry and disillusioned, I did not understand his attitude; as I had never seen him that way before.

He was always patient and had a very good bedside manner. Any way the loose bowel actions stopped and I did end up passing my final examinations. I saw him after my graduation; he was his usual self again when he congratulated me on my result. I could not resist asking him if he recalled why he had spoken to me so harshly. He replied that "of course I remember; I had to stop you worrying quickly as you were so close to your final examination". So I figured that you would stop worrying if you were to get angry with me. It did work so well; he was very experienced and he did know me well; he knew how worried I was about my finals..

I do respect such good physicians that really know their patients and take the time to treat them according to their needs. Now a day, when I get several loose bowel actions, I know the reason for the loose bowel motions; I heed the warning that I am behind with my court reports and I do something about my being stressed- (if I can).

During my final year of medicine we had our first child. I chose an obstetrician that impressed me as one of my teachers. He was always immaculately dressed and wore a college tie. We visited him in his rooms in Collins Street in Melbourne for my wife's antenatal visits. His clientele included the upper class of Melbourne's women. At that time weight increase during pregnancy was of a concern. At one visit, Evelyn had put a on a lot of weight. I did know why she had put on so much weight during her pregnancy; we used to go for a walk every afternoon. Her pregnancy craving with that pregnancy was for chocolate. We could not go past a milk bar; as they were called then; and not go in to get her a chocolate bar. That was not as bad as the her pregnancy craving that she had with our third child-it was an onion; she did not put on so much weight but her breath stunk.

The doctor's waiting room was very formal, so imagine the other ladies when the doctor (obstetrician) came out of his examination room when he finished examining Evelyn. He shouted to me, across the waiting room "Roberto you Locke the fridge". Evelyn nearly died from embarrassment as everybody was looking at her in the formal waiting room. It was so unlike him to behave that way but it worked like a charm. Evelyn did not put on any more unwanted weight for the rest of that pregnancy. Again that was a behaviour from a very experienced specialist to treats his patient in the best and an effective way. That was a lesson that has been invaluable throughout my many years of practice. The rest of the pregnancy was uneventful. She had a long labour of twenty-four hours and delivered our first child, a healthy baby girl. She had a wonderful private room at St Vincent Hospital because I was training there at that time. Women; at that time did stayed in hospital for one week; after their confinement. Evelyn was still in hospital when she delivered our first child Susanne; I was to graduate only a few days later. The specialist, being my one of my teacher, knew of my graduation so he arranged for my wife to attend my graduation ceremony even though it was only several days after her prolonged confinement. He even arranged for her to have a pillow to sit on. She sat throughout the whole of the ceremony in spite of being so sore.

CHAPTER ELEVEN

———— ◆))• •((◆ ————

I graduated from Melbourne University Medical School with an M.B.B.S. in 1969. The MBBS stands for Bachelor of Medicine and Bachelor of Surgery. It was a truly a proud moment to walk up to the podium to accept my hard earned degree. It was great for me after so many years and so many interruptions along the way. It was even more touching to have Evelyn and my parents present at my graduation.

The Melbourne University medical course was so comprehensive and good that after graduating, I could go straight into practice right away but I chose to get further experience before going into practice. I applied for more training at a teaching hospital. After graduating, I did a brief locum while I was waiting for my hospital placement. My placement came up to the Geelong hospital. This hospital was a regional hospital a so I was disappointed because it not a major city hospital. However my disappointed soon evaporated; when I started my residency because the specialists at Geelong Hospital were so good. I did two years internship at Geelong hospital, first as a junior resident and then as a senior resident. The specialist at Geelong hospital knew that I wanted to go to a mission hospital after my placement so they prepared me well with the skills that I did need. They gave me plenty of obstetric, tropical medicine, anaesthetic and major surgical experience.

At a recent reunion of my graduation year, the general feeling expressed by all the graduates that a lot of the training we received both at Melbourne University and the teaching hospitals was wasted as general practitioners. We were trained to do most things; however we often don't get access to hospital beds in major hospitals; to be able to practice the skills we have been trained to perform. I can understand the hospitals now face so many complaints and litigations, with the result they demand a specialist degree to access of their facilities; it does means that a lot of our training has been wasted as we can't practice a lot of the things that we were trained for. Mind you very many the graduates of my year were specialists or the heads of departments, all over the world.

At the Geelong Hospital my hours were horrific; they consisted of one hundred hours one week, alternating with eighty four hours the next week. We did have a room in the hospital to sleep in when we were on call; I was so tired on some nights that after a night calls, I would go back to sleep still holding the telephone. The wards man would have to come up to my room to take the telephone out of my hand to hang it. I don't know how it was that we did not make many mistakes. I will always be grateful to the experienced charge ward sisters that checked our orders and ensured that we did not make mistakes' they often guided us. Research nowadays indicates that working such long hours equates to being badly inebriated so I am very grateful that we did not make some dreadful mistakes. I really don't know how Evelyn managed during that time. We had two young children (babies) only thirteen months apart. One night after I completed a horrific shift I went straight to bed. During the night Evelyn woke up with renal colic. The second child was a vomiter, and so he required a lot of attention. My wife often forgot to drink enough fluids and so she was even more prone to renal colic's. I am not proud of that night; when she could not go to sleep because of her terrible pain I just did give her pain relief and told her to just go back to sleep. The pain did not subside so we eventually had to go to hospital with the renal colic; she had a urinary tract infection as well. If you have ever suffered with renal colic let alone a bad urinary infection you would understand the pain she must have been suffering with. She needed extensive antibiotic intravenous treatment before her pain settled.

I am just as disgusted with myself of what I did to my wife on another occasion. When she finally got to bed she was quite exhausted; Robert would only sleep briefly; he woke up shortly after Evelyn got him to sleep he started crying I cocked up my leg and pushed her out of bed; she did forgive me because I was half asleep; any way it is a dreadful thing to. Somehow and we got through that time.

Late one night I was attending to a dying Catholic patient when he requested that he wanted a priest to give him the last right. I called for the local Catholic parish priest. Evelyn had told me that she has seen that the new parish priest at St Mary's that it was a Father Saul. I did not register, at the time, that it may have been the same headmaster that had expelled me. I did know that if a Christian Brother wished to be a priest at a mature age; he had to go to USA. There was not a seminary for a late vocation in Australia.

So many things had happened since leaving school that I had not given it a second thought.

When the priest came in the middle of the night he recognized me immediately He Exclaimed "you are not a doctor are you!?"

I did not take offense at his comment because I felt vindicated that I had got him out of his warm bed at 2am! I invited him to come to dinner on my day off. My best school friend happened to be in Geelong at that time, so I invited him to come for dinner with our old headmaster. As it so happens my old school friend is the godfather of my second child. I had never heard him say what he said when I told him that our old headmaster would be there. Needless to say he declined the invitation.

I happen to be the medical resident when I was called to a diabetic lady in the Hospital women's ward. Her blood pressure had dropped to a dangerously low level because she had been given a large dose of insulin; her potassium level also fell as a result of the insulin dose. Her potassium was so dangerously low that she could have caused a cardiac arrest. Because it was 3am, I did try but I could not raise anyone for advice. Left to my own devices, I hooked her onto an ECG machine, and then I cautiously started to inject intravenously potassium. Too much potassium can be just as dangerous as too low a potassium level and it can result in a cardiac arrest. I carefully watched the ECG tracing, as the tracing was closer to normal I stopped injecting, as the tracing became abnormal because of the very low potassium, I started to inject again. I kept this up until early morning.

At 6 am the medical physician specialist arrived at the hospital. He told me this practice was very dangerous and I should not have done it. He ordered a blood test of the potassium level, which was only slightly raised. I did ask him what I should have done but I did not get a reply. In any way the lady was very appreciative that I had attended her all night and that she was perfectively well.

My major interest was in the mental health area, so when a specialist Psychiatric teacher; that had been the director of the Victorian Mental Health Service before coming to Geelong Hospital offered to help me to explore mental health. I did think that it was that was a golden opportunity and it could not be missed; so I jumped to accept his invitation. Even though weekends off were so rare and it would mean that the family would miss out; I eagerly packed a bag on a Friday night that I was off for the weekend; and I went over to his house. I was very keen and looking forward to immediately learn all about mental health. Silly me; as a doctor, we never stop learning about mental health problems. As soon as I got there I started to ask him questions; he immediately stopped me and told me "to wait, as Friday night was family night, he would then speak to me. He said "we would now have some family time; then we would have a meal together". On Saturday morning, I keenly expected to learn more, so I asked "if now was the time" he again told me "not now" as he had to take his sons yachting. On our return, I again asked "is it now the time", but again he told me "not now" as we have to wash down the yacht, I don't now remember the sort of yacht it was. I did help his children to wash down the yacht. I was frothing at the mouth so as soon as we got back from washing the yacht I asked him "is the time now?" He told me "not now", we now have to have a BBQ lunch and then afternoon rest. One Saturday evening I again asked and again and again "is it the time now?" I was told "not now" as it was again a family time. On Sunday morning it was church time and so on it went. By Sunday evening I was frothing at the bit and very restless, I had to be back at the hospital for duty soon so I asked impatiently, "when do I get a chance to speak to you and learn about psychiatry? After all that is why you invited me over and you know how scarce weekend off are and I neglected the family to come here!" He replied quite amazed "You have experienced what a family does". Then the lights came on.

He continued, "If you really want to go into psychiatry please keep in mind that what is normal for one person, could well be abnormal to another person". You have just experienced firsthand what one family does at weekend. I will always remember to this day this really invaluable lesson that I learned. It is very important not to be judgmental in any way but to be very familiar with what is a patient's normal life is comprise of.

A (surgical) specialist invited me to go onto his yacht for a sail around Corio bay. Although I do get very sea sick, the weather was quite calm so I decided to take up his offer. I wish I hadn't because during the night a big storm blew up in Corio bay. I spent all the whole night being very sea sick, and fighting back the nausea. In the morning I staggered up on deck to get some fresh air. The experienced sailors were having a beer; they invited me to have breakfast. They told me that if I had a raspberry jam sandwich I would feel much better. I believed them but I did ask why. They replied, laughing loudly, "it will taste the same going down as it does coming up". With that comment I could no longer control the nausea. So over the side I lent and vomited profusely; I could hear them all laughing at me.

During the time at Geelong Hospital many things happened some were quite funny and some were not so funny. The first thing I will relate occurred soon after my second child was born while I was at Geelong hospital; he was supposed to be overdue but he was quite premature. To boot, he was constantly vomiting, He is still very active and he only has 'cat naps'. Today I would diagnose him with having ADD. He is now an adult and he still does he does fit the criterion for an adult ADD; he has learnt many ways to manage the condition. For an example he has learnt to concentrate by tuning out to many inputs. He often manages to sleep four to five hours at night only. When he was an infant, Evelyn consulted a paediatrician for his activity and his constant vomiting. She would feed him for twenty minutes and he would then vomit for the next thirty minutes. She constantly smelt of rancid milk. Naturally he failed to thrive (as we would now call it). The Paediatrician did prescribe some medication for him. Evelyn was very reluctant to give such a young baby any medication. She was so exhausted that he told her "either you give the child the medication or you take it yourself". So she decided to take some medication herself. It only did help a little, but it was not enough so Evelyn had to relent and give the baby some medication. The anxiolytic it did nothing for both the activity and his vomiting; it did nothing for his sleep. Reflux is treated effectively nowadays with reflux medicines. Hyperactivity uses stimulates; exceptionally, for such a young baby

I will discuss the effective treatment of ADD as it is now called, in a latter chapter. When I was on duty I lived at the hospital so one night, the newlyweds was hoping to stay in my room at the hospital. Evelyn came with our 4 months old baby daughter in her bassinet. My daughter started crying soon after getting into my room. I suppose it was a strange place for the child; she had not been there before. Her cry got louder and louder as time went on. We tried everything to pacify her but nothing worked; she just would not be pacified. I am not proud of what we did next. I decided to give her a small dose of an antihistamine; (promethazine) that usually acts as a good sedative with young children. Instead she became very giggly and no matter what we did she would not settle. So finally Evelyn had to leave, that that put our plans to rest.

My Volkswagen (Beetle) died; I decided to take the motor out and recondition it. I would work on the motor in my room at the hospital or in the lounge room in our hospital flat. The lounge room in our flat did have the only gas fire so in the freezing weather in the Geelong's winters it was the only warm place to work in. Even though it was to Evelyn's disgust, I would work on the car there. When I was at the hospital and I had a chance, I took the motor there and I would work on it there; I would try to keep my hand clean by wearing vinyl gloves; in case I was called to a hospital ward; however they rarely did work as they would often break. I am only a bush mechanic; so I broke the oil pump getting it off the motor! I priced a new one, but it was too expensive. So I thought I would try to repair it, I glued it with it with araldite. It actually worked, but I don't know how long it lasted. Anyway, when I got all the motor back together and I put it back into the car. I then got a long time school friend; the one that refused to come to dinner with our old school's headmaster; to help me to try and get the car started.

We towed the car up and down the street but it would not start. So I took the motor out of the car again and took the motor apart again. Naturally I took it back into the lounge room; wife's objected again! I did find out that I had put the crankshaft back into the motor the wrong way round, the front of the shaft was at the back of the motor. When I put the crank shaft back in the right way; when we towed the car this time; the car started right away.

I kept the car for a several years and the oil pump that I had stuck with araldite continued to be ok. I don't know if the oil pump did eventually break down.

As the family was growing and a bigger we bought a bigger car as we could afford one. I think it was a Ford Falcon. By the way petrol cost one shilling and 8 pence a <u>gallon</u> then.

During my casualty rotation, a young girl of sixteen was referral by a local G P. The referral said she was constipated; the general practitioner requested that we should give an enema. My earlier training demanded that we must always do our own examinations so I did do my own examination. Lo and behold, as I examined the abdomen, I felt what felt like a baby kick me; I was sure about my findings when the girl started with contractions. The head was fully engaged so she was ready to deliver her baby.

It was protocol to the telephone the GP that had referred the patient. When I did call the GP, he told me "I could not possibly right". The mother over heard my conversation so she came rushing in and also told me I could not possibly be right; and that her daughter could not possibly be pregnant. In any case, she had to be taken to the labour ward; there she soon delivered a healthy baby girl; in spite of not having had any ante natal care. It says a lot for having children when we are young contrary today's fashion of waiting till the mid-thirties to start a family. When the GP came to visit his patient he went passed me with his head hung low and he did not say a word.

It was very funny when this very psychotic lady came into a very busy casualty. Geelong is a very busy town on a Saturday during summer or the football season; with football injuries and traffic accidents as well all the other problems. The casualty looked like a war zone so one of the senior residents was called to help us in casualty. He was quite arrogant and he thought he knew everything, so the junior residents had nick named him Jesus Christ. Just as the senior resident (that had been called to help us) was coming down the stairs to casualty; this psychotic lady was brought in. The lady was only wearing a nightly; when she spotted him she threw off her nighty, threw herself on the ground and called out loudly 'Jesus Christ!' You can just imagine the laughter that emanated from the junior residents at that time. I don't think he knew why we were laughing so much. The story does not end there; back then we used a terrible drug called paraldehyde to sedate agitated patients. It gives to the patient really bad breath; even though I had used a double dose to try and sedate her, it did not even touch her. As I did not want to use any more, I called the consultant; he told me to put her in a strait jacket and arrange for her admission to a psychiatric hospital. I was also to arrange for an escort to go with her in the ambulance to the psychiatric hospital.

We placed her in a strait jacket. A nurse was chosen because she an especially was a big person. Apparently on the way to hospital she got herself out of the strait jacket; I really don't know how one gets out of a straight jacket. The ambulance had to stop and get some help to restrain her again. They did eventually get her to the Mental Hospital. When the poor nurse returned she was all bruised. I Recently I met 'Jesus Christ' at a medical reunion; both he and his wife are still much the same; they were full of how they were involved in important research; at the same meeting I did meet the director of their research unit. My wife did know many of that years graduates as she was at the Royal Women's Hospital at the same time; she too came to the meeting as she was interested to see what has eventuated with those graduates; we were both amazed at how many graduates of my year are now professors, specialists and head of departments, and they are spread all over the world.

Getting back to Geelong Hospital casualty; on most school days a particular eight year old boy would come into casualty. He was always complaining of various different problems. After checking him out, I would tell him that I could not find anything wrong with him and that he should go to school. He would then tell me "you know I am mentally retired" I think he actually meant to say 'I am mentally retarded" but he was in no way retarded, he just did not want to go to school, I wonder now if he suffered from school phobia; but I knew nothing about that then. I do wonder now if that was the first case of school phobia that I did see and I did not treat it correctly.

When I was working in the outpatient department, several things happened. Some were quite funny others were sad but they are all worth mentioning.

A couple came to consult me because of the problem that actually related to the man's wife. She refused to go shopping in town because she did not trust public toilets. This really restricted their lifestyle. They could not even go shopping together. Any way I suggested that he should get a Porta-Loo and a toilet and put them on a trailer behind his car so that she would always have her own private toilet. I actually said it as a lame joke at the time. At the next visit he thanked me profusely as my suggestion had worked so well. She has never had to use it. I did think in hindsight what it would be like to exit the car and go unto to the trailer; in full view of everyone, to use a toilet; but then again she never had had to use it.

Another incident I recall was in the outpatient waiting room. It very crowded and every department was behind time, so I was called up to help. Just as I arrived in the outpatient department a sister yelled out from across the room "you made me pregnant!" You can just imagine the looks I got! As it so happened, this nursing sister had been trying for quite some time get pregnant. She suffered with a chronic middle ear infection and it was because of the ear infection that she tried but she could not have any success getting pregnant. I suggested that she try an antibiotic that had been written up in a medical magazine. It was often effective in chronic ear infection caused by bacteria called Pseudomonas. This bacterium is sensitive to this antibiotic. The antibiotic's trade name is called Ciprofloxin; we have to get an authorization to prescribe it on the NHS. Apparently she did get a prescription for it from her specialist. She did use it and the result was that her ear infection cleared up and so she did get pregnant. That is why she felt that I was the cause of her finally getting pregnant. As beautiful gesture she called her child Robert after me.

This elderly lady came into hospital emergency room in November; she came into the hospital with symptoms indicating that she needed an operation. On this particular occasion I admitted her suffering with severe abdominal pain. When the specialist saw her, he diagnosed that she had a leaking abdominal aneurism. This is a serious condition and it requires a major operation. As young residents should do, I looked up her history. It was not until I reviewed her case then that I discovered that she presented to the emergency room every November to have a major operation. I discussed her case with that surgeon; he that was sure of his diagnosis but as it was not his field; he told me (but I was sure it only to appease me) that I should discuss the case with a psychiatrist; I did consulted with a psychiatrist that I really respected. He was very interested in my findings; so he advised me to postpone the surgery. That caused quite a furore, if it was in fact a leaking aneurism the surgery was urgent, so the surgeon kept on saying to me "if she dies from the aneurism it would be on your head".

The bed in intensive care was booked just in case the surgery went ahead

Luckily the psychiatrist did back me up and so the surgery was postpone. It was a really stressful time for me! The psychiatrist told me it that I should administer a truth drug intravenously and then question her while she was under the influence of the medication. I think the medication was called Brietal. I was very nervous and not experience in this technique so I asked him to help me. I slowly intravenously injected the drug (under his supervision). She initially started sobbing and then it built up to a cry that we could not comfort her. The psychiatrist told me to very slowly increase the dose. As I did so, ever so slowly, she started to tell us her very sad story. During the big depression, her husband could not get work, so she got a job at a hotel as a domestic. One day, (that she wanted to forget) she was unexpectedly on a 'broken' shift; so she decided to go home and catch up with her washing as her husband had agreed to do the washing but he had not got round to do it yet. When she arrived home she discovered her husband in bed with her very best friend so she immediately left. It was not only very traumatic to find her husband being unfaithful, but to find him with her best friend was too was too much for her to bear. On top of it all she had gone to work to help her family financially. She went to a park and was there for several days, she did not know how long she was in the park for as she was in a trance like state. She does not really recall what went on in the park or even if she ate anything. It was there that she met this very caring lady; she took her into her home and started her eating. There she met her son who was really just as caring. She eventually married the son. She has not known her own mother so this lady became like her own mother; she found what real love was like with her. They lived in a coastal country town; they did not have a resident doctor in the town. Her 'mother' got a cerebral (brain) tumour so the doctor from an adjoining town came to visit her. Because the doctor was not from the town he taught this lady to administer the morphine injection for her 'mothers' pain. As her mother's tumour progressed she became more paranoid. In her confusional state, the mother in law started to accuse her of trying to kill her. This was especially so when she was in pain and the lady had to give her an injection. It so happened that soon after she gave her an injection for the pain the elderly lady died. As a result she has never been able to get over the guilt feelings. Did she in fact kill her? It happened in the month of November. So every November she would come to hospital to be punished by a major operation, (as it were!).

She could not have been able to consciously talk to anyone before about this occurrence (without the aid of the drug). This was because her emotional pain and guilt feelings were too intense. The psychiatrist arranged for her to have several therapeutic counselling sessions. He also invited me to be an observer to these sessions. These sessions were quite intense. He very gently confronted her with what we had learnt under the influence of the drug. He proceeded to explain why she had never been guilty of killing her 'mother'. He carefully and medically explained that her mother's condition meant that her time had come. Her 'mother' was in a lot of pain and was irrational because of the brain tumour and she did need her to give her the injections to relieve the pain. Thanks to the injection she died peacefully. It was total coincidence that she died soon after she gave her the morphine injection. She obviously needed the injection then because she would have been in such pain. The brain tumour was getting worse and it was that that finally killed her. The tolerance to morphine increases as time goes on; so the patient does require a bigger dose for adequate relief of pain and the interval between injections get shorter. Her' mother' was indeed very lucky that she has learnt how to give her the pain injections when she needed them. He explained that most brain tumour are associated with terrible headaches, these can be especially bad when lying down. Again he emphasized that it her 'mother' was so lucky that she had learnt how to give her such relief when she was suffering. The pain in her abdomen eventually settled. She and her husband were both very happy as they went home and I never saw her again.

Now a day's, in palliative care, there is such a thing as a syringe driver that allows the patient to give themselves more pain relief as they do need it.

I learnt how important confidentiality is. We had a lady who came into hospital because of a first trimester miscarriage. In those days, a miscarriage meant a dilatation and curettage to remove any product from conception that was still in the uterus. I administered the anaesthetic for a simple D&C (dilatation and curettage). A senior resident did the operation. At the completion of the procedure, my senior colleague and I were leaving the building. A very concerned husband asked my senior how his wife was, and what was the procedure that his wife had undergone? The second year doctor reported that she was ok and it was only a curette for a first trimester miscarriage, the husband then said "but I have been away for five months".

The woman sued the hospital and the doctor; as the doctor had broken her rights of confidentiality. Never ever give the detail of confidential information out, even to a close relative or partner without first getting permission from the patient. No matter how innocent an enquiry may seem to be at the time. It is of the utmost importance to maintain confidentiality.

Confidentiality laws can however be conflicting. In a life or death situation, confidentiality would not be the first priority for me, and many of my colleagues.

Consider this example before leaving Australia for New Guinea the patient had some blood tests. A doctor gets a call from a doctor in New Guinea; the doctor says my patient in New Guinea and unconscious with cerebral malaria (and so he is unable to give permission for his file to be released) he wants the results of the blood tests.. In the first place we are unable to be sure of what the privacy laws are in that country, secondly we don't know that the patient is really unable to give permission, thirdly and we can't confirm that it is a doctor who wants the information so we don't know how the information will be used. After all it is a phone call. In such a case, most doctors would accept that in a life and death situation they would provide the information.

You can see how vulnerable doctors are if we are duped. When I was in general practice in Kallangur I was called by a solicitor telling me that a subpoena had been issued for my records, as the case was to go to court the following day they wanted the information urgently, the solicitor also indicated that he was acting for my patient. I was in the middle of a very busy evening so he really caught off guard. I did facsimile the records however my records are purposely very difficult to read so he wanted me to translate them for him. The next day I found out that I had been duped. To make matter worse I found out that the solicitors were for the opposing side of the patient. I called the Law Association and my medical defence association. Both were unable to do anything because the senior solicitor said he witnessed the phone call and denied everything that I said the junior solicitor had said to me. Although Evelyn witnessed the telephone call, she was not considered to be an independent witness. I don't know how a senior solicitor from the same office can be called an independent witness.

You would expect that solicitors would respect the law and not lie. I did tell the patient as I related to her the incident and that I had not revealed any sensitive information. She was naturally upset that I had been duped so easily; I lost that patient and I never saw her again.

Returning now to Caboolture outpatients; I did learn another valuable lesson when a very distraught lady saw me. She told me that one night her husband brought her best friend home, he then asked her to move out of the bedroom. He then took the ladies girlfriend into the bedroom. He closed the door and then proceeded to make sounds that indicate that he was having sexual relations. I said "you should not put up with that and you should leave him! " I saw her a few weeks later after her suicide attempt. Only then did I ask to interview her daughter and husband. I then found out that it had been a set up. He really loved his wife, she had been sexually assaulted and raped as a teenager and continued to hate sexual intercourse. In spite of his patience, she did not seem to overcome her dislike of close affection and sexual intercourse and she refused to go to any counselling. So in desperation he confided his dilemma with her best friend. She helped him to devise a plan to shock his wife out of her problem. Her devoted husband and her best friend planned to shock her by getting her to believe that they were having an affair. They believed that shock had to be severe if it was to work. They did not realize that it just would never work. Her emotional damage would only be aggravated by their plan. What a shock that must have been!

To make it worse an inexperienced doctor "me" gave her directive advice and told her to leave him. The depression that followed meant I nearly lost her if it was not for her vigilant only daughter. I learnt that I should never give direct advice, even when I think I know the real facts. Always err on the side of safety. If one is not sure one must get further advice from a more experience doctor.

Many patients do seek direct advice, it is probably ok with purely medical problems to give the options by direct advice but it is dangerous to give directive advice with psychiatric problem. When she found out that it was an attempt by her loving and faithful husband and her best friend to try and help her, she was very relieved and she reconciled with her husband and her loyal friend. It must have works a little because she then attended counselling to help her get over her past sexual abuse. I was so happy everything worked out.

I can give you many examples of the Child Protection Agencies overreacting, when an accusation is made that a parent, usually the father or step father, is sexually abusing their child. The older a child get's more aware that they are believed first and do sometimes make accusations to get out of home or to avoid limits that they don't like. Child protection laws are more like French laws that you have to prove yourself innocent and not like our laws that you are innocent until proven guilty.

I was involved with a number of cases where a teenager made accusations that the father has sexually abused them. In some cases the estranged mothers even supported the teenager. Some cases went all the way to court. Thankfully more often than not the teenager confessed that they had made up the accusation but it is many times at the last moment in court after the caused has spent a lot of money or stress dealing with the alleged accusation. I have also come across some terrible cases of child abuse. I know it is better to protect our children even if it means some innocent men are accused wrongly; hopefully as we get better at this we won't put innocent men in goal.

Back when I was a resident day; one of the resident doctors was to get married. I bet he wished he never had his buck's night at the residents' quarters. We plastered his arms straight so he could not bend his elbows, then we then filled him up with drinks and then we slipped a diuretic in one of his drinks (a diuretic makes you pass urine quickly). We then all laughed at him as the poor man could not reach his fly to undo his pants and pass his urine. He was literally bursting before we took pity on him and removed the plasters.

I was so thrilled that he wanted me for his best man even after what we did to him.

He was Malaysian and he was marring a Methodist girl. In those days I needed permission from the parish priest to enter another denomination church. So I dutifully went to get the permission of my parish priest (that was before Father Saul). I wish that I had not gone to see the priest. After he heard my request, he got quite emotive; he pointed his index finger at my face he shook it and stated "if you as much as step into that church I will excommunicate you". I was flabbergasted. After all it was another Christian church. I was so irate that I just had to talk about it. So I discussed it with the hospital Chaplain. He was an Irish priest and I expected him to be very traditional so I expected him to side with the parish priest. He said to me "let me tell you a joke". I asked "how can that possibly help?" He insisted, and he continued "A Pope died and he went to Heaven, at the Pearly Gates Peter met him. He said God told me to greet you and to let you know everything you want to know about paradise. He told me you have been a very good man". He went on "let me show you around so hop into my limousine". They drove for ten minutes; the Pope kept on asking Peter "what is that high brick wall on our left about?" Peter kept on telling him "just don't worry about that". He took him to the first location. It was a beautiful beach. It had soft sand, breeze and surf. The pope said "this is very nice but I am old now and can no longer surf as I did in my younger days, so what else have you got." Peter said "hop in" As they were travelling to the next place the Pope noticed that the tall brick wall was still there, so again he asked "what is that brick wall is about?" Peter again told him "just don't worry about it". The next place was a peaceful forest scene it had a gentle breeze, lots of birds singing, the smell of freshly cut grass and lots of trees. The

Pope though this will suit me. He then protested to Peter, God told you to tell me everything I wanted to know about paradise. Now listen Peter "what is that tall brick wall about". So Peter said "if you must know it is there for you Catholics, you think you are the only ones here." We all burst out laughing aloud. With that I realized he was a long way ahead of his time and not as traditional as I first though. My wife went to see him because we wanted permission for some form of contraception and the rhythm method was too difficult with my work. He said it is not like you won't have any more children -your health is not good at the moment so it is for health reasons that you need a rest.

Anyway let's now return to the marriage reception. I did go to it. By nine o'clock everyone was very intoxicated. This was a Methodist reception so I thought that they would not consume alcoholic drinks. I asked the caterers what they were serving. "It's only apple juice" the waiter replied. So I asked him to show me the bottle. He brought back an apple cider bottle. It was a Strogbow alcoholic cider, it was cider all right but it contained seven percent alcohol. No wonder everyone was plastered.

During my time in orthopaedics, I would help out in outpatients. I saw a patient that reported that he had been suffering with terrible back pain. It was before the advent of MRIs and multi slice C/T scans were developed, so we had to rely on clinical examination. The patient presented with a terribly bad back. He had been on workers compensation for a bad back for some time so workers compensation asked to make appointment for a review of his back condition. I examined very him carefully. I believed he had a disk lesion. He entered the examination room very slowly leaning heavily on a walking stick and he had a pained look on his face. The examination showed he had limitation of straight raising. He showed numbness just above his left ankle on the outside of his left leg. His back was tender to touch especially on the lower back and on the spines of his lower lumbar vertebra. I presented his case with all my findings to my unit honorary. He seemed to be so disinterested in my findings, he just told me to come to the window and look at the man twirling his walking stick while walking to his fishing boat. It was the same man that so convincingly demonstrated that he had a disc lesion. It was so easy to fake a bad back although experienced practitioner's often would know the fakes. The honorary then explained how difficult it was to detect real back problems. He went on with examples of men that did have real back lesions that were disbelieved because of these charlatans. He then added that he would write the report to Workers Comp and notify them of what we had just seen from the window

The advent of good; multi slice C.T scans and MRI have made this situation much better. None the less some mistakes still do occur, but these mistakes are much less frequent now.

I got great training in general medicine, emergency medicine, tropical medicine, paediatrics, general surgery, vascular surgery, orthopaedic surgery, anaesthetics, ENT, neurology, obstetrics and gynaecology, and of course psychiatry. I don't think I left anything out.

As I have previously stated, the specialist knew what I wanted to do go to the mission hospital in TPNG (as it was then known) after I did finish my further training. So they gave as much experience as they could. They gave me extra experience with surgery, obstetrics and tropical medicine.

CHAPTER TWELVE

After two very educational years in 1970; first as a junior resident then a senior resident at Geelong hospital, I got a job at a Catholic mission in Rabaul. The mission was at Vunapope on the island of New Britain in the Territory of Papua New Guinea. Vunapope is some 40 kilometers from Rabaul and it is very close to Kokopo. At that time it New Guinea was still a Territory of Australia. I had two children by the time that I went to New Guinea. The youngest son was thirteen months old and weighed just twelve pounds and he had started to walk. He was a handful both medically and behaviourally. Thankfully the older child was a dream, she was only thirteen months older than him, but she was already toilet trained and was well behaved.

We booked the flight with the now defunct Ansett Airways to Port Moresby via Cairns. My parents had a fit when we told them that we were leaving to go to TPNG and we were taking the children with us. I did not want to pay excess baggage so I wore the heavy Melbourne jacket and filled all my pockets with my heavy text books. In Australia and the northern hemisphere January is very hot and humid. New Guinea is near the Equator. The flight was via Cairns in Northern Australia so we spent a day there. In Cairns my hands were so swollen from the heat that I thought to myself; how in the world can I do any surgery with my hand like this? When I got to New Guinea I took my heavy Melbourne type jacket and the swelling in my hands settled down so everything was alright. We first had to organize my registration in Port Moresby for TPNG. So we went there first.

The mission had already booked us into a hotel in Port Moresby; so we went there. We went to the reception desk' a pompous man greeted us and found our booking. It was up some stairs and on the first floor. The reception clerk called out to a native busily scrubbing the steps "hey boy takes their luggage to their rooms". We told him that we only had hand luggage so we really could take it too our rooms ourselves and any way he could of seen that for himself. He then directed us to where our rooms were. We started up the stairs; half way up we tried to go round the native that was scrubbing the stairs; the reception clerk saw us; he yelled the poor man in no uncertain manner get out of their way and do take them to their room then start from the beginning of the staircase.

What a culture shock that was! If that is what colonialism is going to be like; we don't want any part of it and we shall have to return to Australia. However once we got out of the capital and into Vunapope we did not find anything like what we saw on our arrival.

On our way to Vunapope; this only a few kilometres from Kokopo, we visited some other Catholic missions. We first called in to an American mission on Buka Island. There we were to meet the Archbishop. Although it was so hot Evelyn was formally dressed with nylon stockings and formal clothing. Obviously meeting an American Archbishop was 'big deal' for us. We greeted what we thought was the Archbishop; the priest told us he was not the Archbishop but told us the man under the 4 wheel drive servicing it was; he would soon come out from under the 4 wheel drive car and would greet us. A man wearing overalls crawled from under the 4 wheel drive car and presented his Archbishop's ring for us to kiss. He was in fact the Archbishop. The rest of the missions were nothing like our first impressions. In fact it put a new beautiful slant on religion. We realized then that it would be nothing like Port Moresby, everyone would be real human and helping each other and the local population. Furthermore it was very refreshing to see the various Missions cooperating with each other. In fact after arriving at Vunapope we were often invited to their (the other Missions) functions.

When we arrived at Vunapope we were greeted by Sister Bernadette. She was an MSC nun. I think MSC stands for Missionary Sisters of Christ,. . Vunapope has a beautiful breeze so my hands were even better. The Vunapope Mission was nothing like we expected. It was like a little town. There were two other nunneries as well as the MSC nunnery, a general hospital, a 'boy's' hospital, a women's section' a pediatric ward, a maternity section, a cook house for the patients' relatives to prepare the patients meals, a private hospital, a dispensary, a nurses' teaching school, a dental clinic and an operating theatre, doctors consulting rooms and a cemetery for those that did not make it.

The rest of the mission had a general store, a power generating plant, a tailor shop, a bake house and a garage complete with a mechanical workshop. There was a Christian Brothers' school for children up to grade six, a mixed race kindergarten and the mission also ran a fleet of ships and boats to supply these outstation; the nuns also provided service to the many 'outstations' they trained the staff to 'man' these stations' and they also provided staff to another hospital that treated T.B. and Leprosy. This hospital was at Bitaparka, across the road from a WW2 cemetery. There were several houses, some for the doctors, some for the priests, some for volunteers, an Archbishop's residency and of course the church. I probably have missed some because like I said it was like a small town on its own.

The mission was very international, there were Australian religious personnel, German bishop, brothers and priests, several nationalities of volunteers from the various trades, and a number of native nuns and brothers. An American order of nuns worked close by and often visited our mission. All the nuns, priests and the Bishop spoke fluent English. I did mention all the heap of volunteers doing all variety of jobs, in their trade. I have mentioned that the mission was very extensive and provided staff for out station as well. They ran a timber plantation to make money to further support the mission.

At the time TPNG was still a territory of Australia and the mission worked with the Australian administration to provide these services.

Vunapope is the local name for the place of the Pope. Soon after we arrived in at the Mission; we attended a ball that had been organized at the Travel lodge hotel to welcome us. At the ball I sky larked with a wig that I borrowed from a lady from a local plantation;

It was quite a fashion for ladies to wear a wig then. Evelyn was very hot and it was as good an excuse as to take her shoes off. She often does anyway.

The next morning we went to the general store. The store manage, (brother) told us that he has heard all about the doctor's wife being so not lady like and taking her shoes off, but he had not heart of my antics. Did it mean that the doctor is excused but his wife is not! She is expected to be a lady at all times?

When we first arrived at Vunapope, we were given a house on the hill overlooking the mission until the doctor's house became available; the doctor I was to replace had not yet left the Mission so we would have to wait to move into the doctor's house. The main doctor's house was a USA army house from WW2. It was made of galvanized iron; the toilet drained into a hole in the sand, the hot water was a large black plastic bag on the roof of the house, the kitchen was separated from the main house by a passage way. It was very comfortable and spacious.

Very soon after we arrived in the house on the hill two native carver ran up the hill and knocked on the door Evelyn answered the door and asked them what they wanted in English; they had two masks that they had carved and that they wanted to sell to her; she liked them both so she bought them both. One was of a mask the other was that of a crocodile. When the men got down the hill they went start to Sister Bernadette and told her that the new lady was 'long long'. That in Pigeon English meant that they thought the lady was mad because she just bought the masks without bargaining with them. Incidentally; many years later we still have; one of the wooden masks with shells for eyes.

I had worked late one night; when I drove back to my house on the hill (before we had moved into the doctor's house) the house was in total darkness; although the mission did have a generator, they did turn it off at 9 pm. After 9 pm we would use battery lights or candle light I left the cars lights on and went into the house. I found my wife and the children huddled on the bed with the mosquito net tightly around the bed. My wife only had a torch. I asked why they were all in bed like that she replied "because a terribly large coconut beetle attacked your small child's big toe and it started hissing". I did tell her that it really would not do them any harm, although they did sound ferocious.

Sister Bernadette had arranged for us to have home help as soon as we moved into the doctor's house; the women home helpers were called 'Marys"

We found that we were going through them as if they were out of fashion.

So we asked Sister Bernadette what we were doing wrong. She explained that Evelyn was working with them so they considered that she was not satisfied with their work. Evelyn would tell them let us wash the mould of a wall and that she would start at one end and the "Mary" could start at the other end. So the "Marys' just got up and left.

My wife told Sister Bernadette that she was not like the other ladies and would not play golf or go to the clubs; so that if she had nothing to do she would go mad with boredom. Sister Bernadette suggested she could instruct the native trainee nurses with their obstetric lessons. My wife agreed to that.

She had two Sepik girls in her group of trainee nurses. One day, she was teaching the girls in our house when a Sepik wood carver came to the door. She asked him to wait until she had finished the lecture; he spotted the Sepik girls and became very upset.

We again learned that we must respect their different cultures; and that with ignorance we could make some dreadful mistakes.

Apparently she was unaware that in the Sepik culture no man has to be kept waiting by Sepik women. Luckily he did make allowances for Evelyn's ignorance of their culture so he just left, but he was very annoyed.

Another interesting fact that is in the New Guinea culture is that women have the right to inherit land; however it is their brother or their nearest <u>male</u> relative that controls the land.

Not long after I arrived the doctor I was relieving went on holidays. So naturally, when this twelve year old girl came to the hospital because of severe abdominal pains the nuns called me. I examined the girl and she was very tender in the right lower abdomen. That amounted to an acute appendicitis. At that time surgery was indicated so I asked the nuns to prepare her for surgery and get the operating theatre ready. One of the nuns was qualified to administer the anaesthetic. When I opener her abdomen up a tape worm greeted me wriggling out her appendix. After removing her appendix and treating her for worms she made a good recovery. I learnt to think about worms in the tropics. .

Soon after I got to the Mission a patient had a heart attack. At the Hospital in Melbourne or Geelong I would start the heart massage and alternate with the artificial breathing, usually there was plenty of help in such an emergency; however at Vunapope I did not have such a luxury, so I stated the massage and yelled at the nurses to get me the oxygen and the suckers. These where not piped as it is in our Hospitals, but the oxygen was in a gas cylinder on a trolley and the suction was a portable unit. After several minutes and no response I got a patient who was watching me to go get my wife. The ward was an open ward not like our modern wards in hospital that allow for privacy. My wife soon came to help me. I asked her to get me the equipment I had asked the nurses to get me. When she went to the cupboard where the equipment was kept she found the nurses hiding there. The patient recovered. After the emergency was over and I found out that I had frightened the native nurses by my yelling to them. So in subsequent emergencies I learned to gently ask the native nurses "You know where the oxygen and sucker are kept now go and get them for me"; then I would return furiously to the patient.

I had a lot of problems with sick children disappearing during the night. Often they were even sicker when they did return. Many had diarrhoea and were on intravenous fluid replacement so when they returned they were even more dehydrated.

I had worked up a good rapport with some of the native mothers; so I asked them what was happening, why was I loosing so many children and that were coming back were even sicker when they did? They told me that the children were being taken to their witch doctor during the night. So I asked them to tell the witch doctor that he was welcomed to come to the hospital; he should avoid being seen by me or the nuns (especially the nuns) and not to interfere with my treatments. He could work his craft on the children in hospital. I never did see him and I never lost a child from then on so it was a win–win for both of us!

While I am on the topic of their beliefs, I do want to talk about a very important belief that the New Guinea natives believe in. They believe that the blood of a labouring woman is cursed. So that when a women starts to bleed during a complication of labour they can't be put her into their vehicle to bring her to a hospital- so they bring them to hospital either too late or not at all and the woman dies! I had to work very hard to dispel that belief in my area, I had to disprove their false belief and prove that blood from a labouring woman did not curse their vehicle I would only be called to the labour ward for the complicated deliveries; the nun- mid wives would deliver the other 1100 babies. They very first native baby that I delivered was not just pale but it was very white. The nun in the labour ward must have seen my intensely surprised expression because she took me aside and told me that all the native babies were born pure white; because they were not exposed to the sun in the mother's womb. They did not become colored until after a few days after their birth; once the sunlight got to them.

I had learnt a common comment in Melbourne at the Women's Hospital that was asked to labouring mothers at the time that they were ready to deliver their baby. I would ask the lady if she wanted to push. So when I was called to a lady that was ready to deliver her baby I asked the lady if she wanted to push; everyone in the labour ward starting to laugh; I asked them why they were all laughing at me; I was told that in pigeon English, it meant did she want to have intercourse! Can you imagine a lady being asked if she wanted have to sex, with the doctor none the less and with everyone watching; at the time of her delivery.

I had been told to never stop the car if there was a crowd on the road. I was on the way back from Bitaparka Hospital, with my family in the car, when I came across a large crowd in the middle of the road. I automatically slowed the car and then stopped. The crowd picked up the Volkswagen and stated to rock it. We wound up all the windows as I felt we were in real trouble. I was soiling the seat, so to speak. It was a truly terrifying experience. Suddenly an elder appeared from nowhere and yelled out to the crowd "he is the mission doctor". We all felt greatly relived as the crowd put down the car and as quickly as they had appeared they disappeared. We later found out that the Tolias were having a fight with the whites. So it was just as well that the old man recognized the mission car and told the villager that I was the mission doctor. I really don't want to think what would have happened if that old man had not been close by and had not recognized the car.

It never did happen to me again as I and my car became better known to the villagers.

My mother in law came to visit. She did not really like the blackish volcanic sand around Vunapope, so my wife decided to take her and our two children, to a friend's plantation round the corner to a bay that has beautiful white sand, like the sand is like on the Gold Coast. As it so happened the Volkswagen had seen better days so the Mission provided me with a new Ford Cortina. On the way my wife got a flat tyre. She tried to change the tyre but the new jack was defective it would not hold up the car up so that she could change the tyre. So there was nothing that she could do except, to get help. The coconut factory was close by; so my wife told her mother to carry one child and she would take other. So they went to the coconut factory to get help. She told her mother not to look at the up at any of the natives.

The Tolias and the Chimbus were having a fight. The natives made improvised weapons like six foot long plank of wood with six inch nails driven through at one end. They could really inflict major injury. I actually saw a man that died after suffering such an injury.

At that time; they left expats along; unless they played around with their women. Incidentally I did hear of a man that had to be flown out urgently because he has been playing up with their women and his bosses became aware that the native were about to kill him.

On the way my mother in-law kept on saying to my wife 'look they don't have clothes on'. Any way the natives did not annoy my wife's party, and she did get to the coconut factory, they came to the car to and changed the tyre for her. My wife then took her mother to the plantation that has the white sand beach.

I will now tell you about some of the other interesting experiences that I had while I was at the Mission Hospital.

A native school teacher had walked for half a day to arrive at Vunapope on a Saturday afternoon. He told me that he has a "fendix". That is a Pigeon English for an appendix. I thought to myself 'sure you walked at least some ten kilometres with terrible abdominal pain'. It did not seem consistent with the fact that he had walked such a distance, with terrible abdominal pain from an appendix infection. I did examine him; sure enough he had all the signs of an acute appendicitis. I asked the nuns to get him ready for the operating theatre.

At the operation, I drained some half a litre of pus from his abdomen, his appendix has certainly burst.

On the Sunday morning when I saw him then next morning following his operation; he seemed to be recovering well. He told that he would have to get back to his class for Monday. Again I thought to myself "no way' after such an infection and surgery."

However that afternoon he was gone. The different levels of pain threshold that our society's patients display are amazing. I have seen patients that only have a splinter yet are almost dying with pain.

At another occasion; a man presented to the hospital because he believed that bad medicine has been worked on him. Bad medicine is similar to what our Aboriginals believe, that "the bone" has been pointed at them. He came to the hospital emaciated, unable to eat and he complained of having a "blocked bowel". He has not eaten for quite a few days so naturally his bowels were in fact empty, but he did worry about his bowels because he was unable to open his bowels. He could not be convinced that he had not been a victim of bad medicine and that was the cause of his problem; but he was dying before my eyes.

So I decided to play his "game"; I told him that I did not know if my medicine was powerful enough, but I would like to try. I stood him in front of my x-ray machine. It was small portable x-ray machine left over by the USA army from WW2. I told him that I would take a picture and if the picture was white then my machine had worked. I had effectively chased out the bad medicine away, however if the picture was black my machine was not powerful enough to chase the bad spirit away. I used a high setting on the x-ray so that it was enough to make the film white. I showed to the patient his x-ray film, he immediately felt ok. He stated eating, and several days later he went home.

I think it was 1971 when an earthquake hit Rabaul; I was operating at the time so I could not stop. When I had finished the operation I went out of the operating theatre onto the wide veranda that was around the theatre. On the veranda there were many patients waiting to be seen. I found out that they were from a highland village school that has sustained a lot of injuries in the earth quake. As I tried to triage the most injured. The nuns told me to go to see the teacher, however I noticed a child that was very quiet, and pale. He was only about six years old. When I did look at him more closely; I found that he has lost the complete pulp of his right heal.

Apparently he was at school when the earth quake happened. The concrete floor opened up and then closed catching and cutting off his heal. I took him immediately to theatre before the shock hit him. I did a pedicel full thickness graft from his other calf.

He lay so still while the graft developed its own circulation so then I could separate the graft and allow his legs to be separate. I had to use every bit of my surgical training and I was so grateful to my teacher at Geelong Hospital. All the other injuries were not so bad.

My wife happened to have gone shopping into Rabaul on that occasion; she was naturally worried when she could not get back because was told the road was closed. To make matters worse she heard that they were expecting a tsunami because Simpson bay is a basin (it is the creator of a large extinct volcano). She finally was relieved; when I finally got a message through to her that I was ok. She and the children, stayed at a friend house in Rabaul that night. She found it very interesting that when she had previously experienced an earth quake while at our Vunapope house, the fridge door and all the cupboard doors opened and discharged all their contents, however the Government house she stayed at; and the occupant of the friend's house were not so tidy; did no such thing. It has been built to sustain such a sway.

Now to a very humorous incident that happened to me while I was there! I was called to a private home, not far from the mission, to see a child in severe pain with an ear infection. I wanted to prescribe an antibiotic for her ear infection but the mother was adamantly against it. The child's mother is a sociologist (I don't know if she is still alive) she has several books to her credit. The girl was eight years old. The mother reassured me that all she needed was breast milk and with that she put her daughter on her tiny breasts. I was trying to be diplomatic and trying hard to avoid the embarrassment that her daughter felt having to be put on the breast, so I explained that she would not have any breast milk. However it seemed to no avail. She refused the antibiotic prescription. The next morning she was at the maternity hospital purchasing breast milk from the native lactating mothers that has just delivered their babies.

"Help us" she writes books giving advice to people; in any case the girl did eventually get better. Recent research using meta-analyses did show that it is unnecessary to use antibiotics for simple ear infections as they eventually get better. If your child wakes up at night with an otitis media (middle ear infection) and is in terrible pain, you will opt for the quicker cure. I must tell you about a very interesting technique that some practitioner used for weight loss. At one stage the Mission got a second doctor; his technique for overweight European patients was to ask them to take all their cloths of behind the curtain; when they were undressed he would open up the curtain and take a Polaroid photograph of them in their birthday suit.. He would say that the patient that did come back effectively lost a lot of weight. I did point out that the large majority never did come back!

We eventually got a lovely a lovely "Mary" as they were called. She was well educated and spoke perfect English. One evening, we had invited some friends over for dinner. When they arrived they spoke to our "Mary" in Pigeon English, she replied to them in Pigeon English, and then she spoke to us in perfect English. You then should have seen our guests' faces. That was not only their only surprise that was in store for them. My wife was cooking beef stroganoff (for our dinner); our younger son thought he would help her so; unbeknown to her he went outside and got a hand full of black sand –grit and added it to the food she was cooking. When it came to have dinner; our guest did not want to be impolite so when it came to dinner they painfully tried to eat the meal; when we started to eat; we realized what had happened. We then stopped them trying to eat the gritty meal and we then found something else to eat. They incidentally became very good friends. They were the managers of the plantation that has the beautiful white sandy beach. We sometimes would play 500 with them; the husband would exclaim to his wife "for goodness sake Rita" when she made a wrong call. That saying stayed with us even till now.

One day we went to their place for dinner; she served a beautiful steak tartar (raw fillet and a raw egg). Because I had been feeling off all day; can you imagine how that meal then was welcomed by me?

I arranged for them to a adoption a baby girl. They did have one son but she was Rhesus negative. In those days it was a major problem so she could not have any more children. This day's a simple injection just after birth has prevented this problem. We still have some contact with that child. We did see them when we and they returned to Australia. They use to have a new year's party every year to which all their friend were invited.

My young son got bacterial diarrhoea, thankfully I had samples of a German antibiotic that was effective with that bacteria. The Mission often got German samples sent to them; some were out of date but none the less effective. The only problem was that this antibiotic (called Anabactyl) was an injection; it was to be given twice daily for 5 to 7 days. My son's buttocks were rather small; as you might recall he was little; to make matters worse he had lost a lot of weight with the diarrhoea. Every time he saw me coming with the injection he would say "no daddy no daddy" and started crying. It must have been very painful especially with his small buttocks. You can imagine how difficult it was to give him the injections! Any way it did cure him. When he did get better; it was great to see this small person running on the beach.

I did have to do some bigger operations, because although the Government hospital did have a resident surgeon; when he went on holidays; Nonga Hospital had an arrangement with the Royal Melbourne Hospital that they would send up a relieving doctor. On one of this occasion the registrar that came up to Rabaul was no better equipped to do the surgery than I was.

One of the American nuns had bowel cancer; she did not want to go back to USA or anywhere else to be operated on. In spite of my insistence of how important her condition was and that she returns to the USA; she adamantly refused to go and insisted that I look after her. So I agreed to do the operation. I removed the localized cancer and gave her a colostomy while the wounds in her bowel healed. I latter repaired the colostomy and returned her normal bowel function. Thank fully all did go well, thanks again to the training that I got at Geelong Hospital. You should have seen me the morning before the operation studding the surgical atlas to refresh my mind and to make sure that I remembered all the steps. As you may recollect that was one of the surgical atlases, that was one of the heavy books I has in my jacket when I first flew to New Guinea.

Although I always on call the hospital was often within easy reach if I was wanted. If I was not in reach the nuns would handle most things and as I said the Government hospital Nonga Hospital was also within easy reach. On some occasions we went to the see some of the caves that the Japanese built during the WW2. These were simply amazing. The openings were not as impressive, but the insides of the caves were fantastic. One was even large enough to take a large barge; another was quite large; it opened up into a huge cave that was a Japanese military hospital. Apparently they forced the local people to help them dig these tunnels. My elder children don't remember seeing the caves; they were only 3 and 4 at the time. I was told that during the war the Australian doctor could not get enough intravenous fluids; so he improvised and used the sterile isotonic coconut milk for intravenous fluids. There were plenty of coconuts available and in this way he saved many lives.

There were many wrecks of crashed airplanes and ships both Japanese and the Allied forces. There were also many unexploded bombs on the island from the invasion of New Guinea. Recently, I saw a news report that the Australian Navy is in Rabaul are disposing the very many unexploded bombs from the war. Evelyn and I were totally unaware that when trekking through the bush that there could have been unexploded bombs.

We used to go through the bush with the nun to native villages to deliver heath information and basic health treatment including immunization for children. On another break we went to the New Ireland. The mission arranged for us to go there on a mission Cessna. That was quite an experience; the scenery was beautiful, even magical; tropical beaches, palm trees, blue sky. It would have been even better if I has not got air sick, to make maters Evelyn laughed at me.

We did go on a Mission boat to visit some outstations; luckily the sea was very calm so I did not get seasick on that trip.

On another break, we visited the site of the Bougainville mines. The landscape was amazing it was so steep. We saw a huge earth moving machine that had fallen down a ravine; it was just left where it lay; it was too difficult and too expensive to get it back out. When we got to the mine we saw a huge Euclid truck. We thought that it would make a good photo if our child was next to the huge wheel of the truck. I took Robert next to the truck; he was terrified by the huge truck wheel so we settled for a photo of me next to the trucks wheel. The wheel was taller than I was.

I do want to repeat we were amazed as to how the different religions cooperated so well with each other. There were so many missions, why is it that they don't seem to tolerate each other as well at home? There are Catholics, Seventh Day Adventists, Church of England, Methodists and Lutherans. I don't think I left any one out. In fact in the Catholic Church the priest; who was not so young; invited different ministers, of the many different Christian faiths, to conduct ecumenical services; at the Catholic Church.

I only had one situation were religion caused me a problem as a doctor. A sixteen year old man young man, of the Jehovah Witness faith was cutting down trees with his father, when a heavy log fell the wrong way and landed on his thigh. It cause compound fractured his leg (the femur). He had lost a lot of blood before the others got him to hospital. He developed a raging infection whilst in hospital so he urgently required a blood transfusion. Because of his religious beliefs he and his parents' refusal to give him the transfusion so I could not give it to him. I did discuss the seriousness of his condition with his parents and that in order to save his life he needed a blood transfusion urgently. (Blood expanders were not available then). The parents could not decide but they tended to agree that that was the only option left to save his life. A church elder kept on coming to visit the very poor and sick man, but his reason was to tell him that he would perish forever if he took the blood.

He needed his badgering like he needed a hole in the head. Finally I got a court order to give him the transfusion and thereby stopping all the hassling. They were not able to tell him it was his decision because he did not have any say in the matter; it was a court order. He recovered well and I hope he lives well into his old age.

At the end of 1972, I had completed my stint at the mission hospital so it was time to return to Australia. The natives have a fruit called a pomello. It is a little like a grapefruit however the flesh inside is pale orange. They cut it in half emptied the flesh in one half and use it as a receptacle. They then use it to collected money to for their cause, in this case to give to me as a send off. When the locals from a village close by found out that I would be leaving soon; an elder from a local village came to the back door of the house to present me with this gift to show the villager gratitude. There was some twenty dollars in the half pomello. A nun happened to be in the house at the time that he presented me with the gift. I started to tell him to buy something for the village children with the money that the village had collected for me. The nun put her hand on my shoulder and whispered to me "you bastard". I stopped immediately saying what I had started to say; "this was a great but perhaps the village and you could buy something for the village children with the money in my memory. I was so surprised hearing a nun saying what she did say that I instead said "thank you so very much for the much for appreciated gift". I spun around as soon as he left and asked the nun why she said what she whispered to me. She told me that I should learn to be humble and that people have the right to please me, as well as I have the right to please them. That was another in valuable lesson that I will never forget. Later we did visit that village; and I discovered that the village looked after a retarded adolescent. After we came to Australia we still kept in contact with that nun, in fact she came to stay with us in Australia at one time. The locals put on a lovely "sing-sing" for our send off. On the way back to Australia we used the opportunity to see some of the New Guinea highlands. That turned out to be some experience. We could have driven to Mt Hagen, but that is the end of the highway, it was quite rough in places and a very busy highway with many trucks using the highway, so we chose to go there by airplane. The mission arranged for us to flight to several of their other Catholic Missions and to be able to stay there. While we were in Mt Hagen we visited a local village there. Sue, our four year old daughter wanted us to get handkerchiefs and undies for the children. They were all naked and they all had to have green pussy discharge from their noses. The whole family, including the pigs, sleep in their hut. It is so cold at night in the highlands that they have a fire all night in their hut. They cover themselves in pig fat to keep warm. The days were quite warm so when the sun came out the smell is horrific; they don't smell it as the nose quickly adjusts to odours.

Waa was our next stop. The only way in to Waa is by aircraft. The weather has to be considered always as visibility can be very limited. Waa lies between two mountain peaks (on each side). The airfield is quite unique; it is actually built on a slope; the planes land uphill to slow them down and they take off uphill so the planes get enough speed to take off. It was really spectacular when the plane approaches the Waa airfield. We wondered how the pilots managed to land their planes onto the airfields between such tall mountain peaks on either side.

On the way we experienced another wonder. We were flying over a dormant volcano. The pilot asked Evelyn if she wanted to see a volcano creator. She agreed so with that, he banked the plane steeply and went right into the creator of the volcano. I was very scared at first, but then the sight was so spectacular that I forgot any apprehension. I suppose he had done this manoeuvre many times before, as he seemed so experienced…. I hope.

The mission at Waa was quite primitive, when compare to Vunapope. They only depended on donations as they did not get any Government subsidy. The natives were so friendly that we mixed freely with them. It was not until later that we read somewhere that not so long ago they were still cannibals. I was also reading an article about a disease that only seemed to affect women's brains; it caused their paralysis and their eventual death. Women are considered to be of even lesser value than their pigs by New Guinea men; certainly in the past. It turns out that when they were still cannibals men ate the good parts of their human prey, the children were next to eat and finally the women had what was left. That was usually was the diseased brain, hence the disease affected mainly women. As the practice of cannibalism is dying out so is the prevalence of this disease dying out. We were at the Catholic Mission in Waa on a Sunday so naturally there was a Mass. A large proportion of New Guinea population in Waa is Catholic; because of the Catholic Mission there. At the finish of the Mass everyone gathered in the church grounds; many of the locals gathered around us. At first I thought they were looking at our children as my older daughter has beautiful blond curly hair. Then I realized that it was my dental plate that they were so interested in. I had been playing with my dental plate during Mass. It turned that they had been looking at me during Mass and they were fascinated by the dental prosthesis. I was able to show them the dental plate. They were also very interested in my wife's glasses. When they tried to look through my wife's glasses they were amazed that she could see anything looking through them, she is very short sighted. We take such things for granted but these primitive natives have never seen anything like these items before.

When we were back at Vunapope; as I explained we had electricity for some part of the day at least. A highland native visited us, I don't recollect the reason now, but I do remember the occurrence. He stood next to the light switch, as he turned it on he looked at the light bulb, he then turned the switch off, he then turned on again and then looked at the light bulb. He kept on doing it for at least five minutes. The look on his face indicated that he was confused - was it magic?

We experienced another highlight while we were on the New Guinea highlands. The cooler climate of the highlands allow a farm to grow fruit. I don't know if that farm is still there. Our children had only ever tasted frozen strawberries; so when my children got a taste of the_fresh fruit they hoed into them. You should have seen them covered in red juice as they ate loads fresh strawberries. Finally we returned to Australia. Australia granted New Guinea independence just before we left New Guinea. Evelyn contends that the then Prime Minister of Australia; at that time must have not have left his hotel room or he would seen how primitive some of them were and that they were not really ready for self government.

Recently I had the opportunity to visit Rabaul. Evelyn and I chose this particular Princess Cruise because it called into Rabaul. It was very interesting to see it again after so many years. Many changes have happened since we had been there well over 40 years ago. The town of Rabaul has moved to Kokopo near Vunapope since the volcano eruption in 1996. The volcano eruption decimated the town of Rabaul; its original airport is now buried under several meters of volcanic ash, the Travel Lodge Hotel that we so many a good times at the; remember the welcoming party? It is covered in ash but it is being restored. The big volcano is called "the mother" and the smaller dormant volcano is called the "daughter". The volcano seems to be constantly rumbling and volcanologists are constantly monitoring the activity of the volcanoes. The 'mother' is active and could erupt at any time. The Travelodge hotel could be buried again if the volcano erupts again. I don't think we would like stay there.

On our return to Rabaul we nostalgically wanted to go return to Mission and see any changes that have happened to the Mission; so we got a local native to drive us back to the Mission. He asked us if we minded if he took his ;8 year old daughter along with us for the drive. It was school holidays as well as a Saturday, so he was looking after his daughter. He spoke really good English. He told us he had gone to private English school till grade 6. We told him that I had been at the hospital many years ago so we were very interested to see it again.

He drove us there in his Ford twin cab. On the way to Kokopo he pointed out his village. It was well kept and very tidy. We were impressed as to how neat it was. I think it was an SDA mission. Even though the road from Rabaul to Kokopo has become very busy as main town has moved to Kokopo and it is now the capital of New Britain.

The sides of the road were unkempt; portions of the road were just dirt as the tar was nonexistent anymore. The dust was so bad and the driver had got us to wind up the windows of the car; along those sections. Apparently, they did not have any rain for over a month; that had made matters worse; Australia still gives New Guinea a lot of money but I don't think it reaches the correct pockets.

He made a stop along the way so that we could get a beautiful view of the volcanoes across the bay. He also made at the stop at the entrances of the Japanese's tunnels. We did see that little has changed in those things since we were there.

When we got to Kokopo the development that has taken place there is amazing. There are several supermarkets, all the banks are represented, there several garages, all of the professionals like solicitors etc. and there even is a post office. He took us to the Mission as I had asked him to. The Mission it is now separate to the hospital. There still is a German Archbishop in the original Archbishop's residence.

The three nunneries were all empty. I don't know where they went; the European (German) nuns probably have returned to their motherhouse, the American nuns have probably found another Mission, the Australian nuns have returned to Australia in their mother house in Sydney. I could not find out where the local nuns went.

I realized that the Mission no longer ran the hospital; so I asked the driver to take us next door to the hospital. He drove us there; he parked under a tree for shade and told us to take our time to see what we wanted to see and he would be there to take us back when we were ready.

I introduced wife and myself to the doctor at the hospital and I told him I had worked there many years ago. Apparently doctors are still being employed from Australia the present one is named Felix. We did read on the notice board that a visiting Australian Orthopaedic surgeon was to visit the hospital in 2 weeks time. The doctor seemed very busy so he introduced us to the officer responsible for hospital hygiene. The health officer then took us round the hospital. The buildings that were "new" many years ago are the ones they are using now. During the time I was there the volunteers built the 'new' hospital wing. As I remember it; it was a large H shaped building. One side of the H had the private ward, the children's ward and the dental clinic; the other part of the H had the doctor's consulting rooms, the x-ray room and the operating theatre, the part in between the sides consisted of the pharmacy and the basic pathology laboratory. I think the private hospital is now the administration centre. The older parts of the hospital have gone; the "cook house" has gone; remember it was the place that the relatives of hospital patients used to prepare the meals for the patients, the boys hospital has gone, the old maternity wards where I attend the complicated deliveries and I think there is no longer a private ward. The general wards are now on that section. The operating theatre and the consulting rooms are still being used as such. We visited the wards, we met the some of the nurses, we saw the brightly painted children's ward and we talked to a few of the patients.

I only saw the operating theatre from the outside but I understand that they are still using it and are using the same equipment. I under stood that they still use the old x-ray machine that I used. It was old back then, so it amazing that it still works. There has been some progress. The wards only had wooden beds when I was there, now they all have simple metal beds.

We meet a volunteer physiotherapist; he was lovely, we did not have that the luxury years ago. Even though there were a lot of "tradies" as volunteers then. The cemetery was the very same that the nuns buried our unborn child; when Evelyn had a miscarriage. There was a fresh grave in the cemetery. The health officer explained that unfortunately a doctor had unexpectedly died. We were not told. Was he In fact killed? The hospital grounds were quite neat and clean but not as pristine as the nuns kept them when we were there.

I think the Mission donated the buildings and the grounds to the New Guinea Government before they left.

Our driver and his daughter were waiting for us; when we returned to the waiting car when we had finished the very interesting tour of the hospital. The driver then drove us back to Rabaul on the way back he offered to drive us to see the Catholic Church in Rabaul; It was not part of our initial agreement but it does demonstrate how obliging and friendly they are. We thought that it really would be interesting. We attended our first Ecumenical service there. When he took us back to the Catholic church everything was the same inside; it was like going back in time as we went back into the church As I sat in one of the church pews memories started to flow back to me. I felt like I was back at mass back in the days long ago. I remembered the parish priest inviting the minister of the Church of the England to deliver a joint sermon. Evelyn remembered how she recalled the minister that did give the joint sermons. When he was teenager; he was a good friend with her 2 brothers. The three of them used to sit at the back of the church and tell jokes and laugh during services. Back then; Evelyn and the minister looked at each other; they immediately recognized each other. He whispered in her ear "if you won't tell neither will I". It was so refreshing to remember that we attend such a service so many years ago. Back it was a truly living Christian experience in the real sense of the word; to witness such a service, it really made religion alive for us.

I remember how a priest (he was an Aussie) used to come to the house in the evenings and ask Evelyn if I had been to mass that Sunday or if I had been too busy. If I had not had a chance to get to a mass, if I had not; he would there and then just say mass for me. These people and the experiences there made religion truly be alive for us. We should not judge religion by its priest or ministers however they do often influence our perception of religion. I also remembered how he would come to our house and ask if he could just use our bed. They were so human and real.

The grounds outside the church were the same except for the black volcanic dust everywhere.

When we finally did get outside of the church, we took a lot of photos including of the driver and his beautiful daughter. The native driver then took us back to the pier where the ship was docked. The natives had a market selling their wares just for the passengers. We did purchase two Buka baskets as or one from many years ago was breaking. The natives were so friendly and happy. As we sailed away so many wonderful memories flowed back to both of us; it was so good that we did make the effort to see to the locals, Rabaul and Vunapope again.

CHAPTER THIRTEEN

———— ◆))·((◆ ————

After our time on the Mission, we returned to Australia. We decided that we did not want to go back to Melbourne's changeable weather; Melbourne weather can change so quickly so that we can have four seasons in one day. It can be boiling in the morning by the afternoon it can be storming, raining and freezing. We experienced a good example Melbourne's weather of when visited my parents in Melbourne some time ago. During that visit, the day was very hot, so we took our children to a swimming pool; by then the older children were teenagers so they could look after the younger children; while we went to visit some friends about half an hour's drive away. The children's objections vigorously, but my wife insisted that the children take some warm clothing with them. When we returned to pick up our children they were shivering, in spite of them wearing all their warm clothing. The weather had changed in a matter of hours, (as Melbourne's weather can).

On another occasion; it was so cold that we were sharing a meal with our old school friends, sitting on a bed in the only room that has a fireplace; it happened to be the maim bedroom.

On the way back, on the way south, from New Guinea I visited several hospitals in North Queensland. There I enquired about several medical superintendent positions with the right of private practice, but they all proved to be not quite suitable for what I wanted.

When I got to Brisbane I had an interview with the Director of Child and Family Guidance a Division of the Queensland Government Health Department (now that Division of Queensland Health is called Child and Youth Mental Health of CYMS for short). Although some people did find the director stern; I found him to be a lovely person. After the meeting with both him and his wife; she too was a qualified child psychiatrist; she ended up being my supervisor; during my early training with that Department, I decided that this was what suited me to the core. I am very interested in the problems that children have, and what their parents' do to deal with them. The department offered further training in just that as well as psychiatric problems. I was offered a position as a medical officer with that department so I grabbed it. The director accepted that I wanted to go to Melbourne to seem my parents and to get our belonging that they had stored for us. So I did go there firs before I was to start with that Department. I first I bought a white Holden station wagon for $28000, and then hired a one way trailer to carry our goods back, (that my parents had stored them for us.)

The director of the Division of Child Guidance had told me to get back as soon as possible to start my new job. We hurried to get everything sorted out in Melbourne; I loaded the trailer hooked on the back of the new car and started on the long drive back. On the way a tyre on the trailer blew out. Luckily we were getting into a town so we were only driving slowly, so I did not lose control of the car or trailer; the only damage was to the goods on the trailer; a big plate at the bottom of a tea chest that we put most of our goods in did break. A very helpful tyre dealer helped us to get a second hand tyre; as we did explain that we were on a tight budget. The rest of the journey to Brisbane was uneventful.

I was driving across the Story Bridge as I got into Brisbane; it was on a Friday. I was listening to the car radio when a news item reported that the Mary Street clinic had just burnt down. That was the place that I was supposed to start work at on the Monday!

I had to wait six weeks before the Department found me a new place to work from; it was the Spring Hill headquarters of the Division. I filled the six weeks by doing locums until the place was ready. I needed a car to do the locums so I bought a 1962 Fiat. The car was quite old but, it was quite cheap, it was good and it served me well for my purposes.

One night at about 11pm I got an urgent call to go for an after-hours home visit. An elderly lady; I think she was about 80 years of age; was having severe chest pain. I should have taken the good car however out habit I took the "work" car. I set off, probably, speeding at 75KPH. The police pulled me up for speeding, when I explained to them that I was a doctor on an urgent call and that I was going to a suspected heart attack. The police replied "Ok mate then follow us". They took off with their light flashing. I tried to keep up but my poor old Fiat could hardly travel past 80 KPH! The police car did some 100 KPH. I did eventually get to her in time and I dealt with her chest pain which was an angina attack, and it all went well. She later had a further attack did have to go to hospital. These days I would not waste valuable time, so I would just get the paramedics and an ambulance to take her to hospital.

On another occasion during those locums, I got a very annoying call early on a Sunday morning; a man had forgotten to get a repeat repatriation prescription on the previous Friday for his constipation medications. He told me he needed that prescription as he had difficulty opening his bowels; he did not tell me the reason he needed the home visit until I had got there. He had initially told me he had severe abdominal pains. I suppose constipation can cause abdominal pain and it can be a major problem for the elderly. I suppose he did try, and did wait till the Sunday before calling me; but he could have waited just a few more hours.

Eventually my appointment to child guidance did take place and I did not have to do these locums any more. The training at the Division of the Health Department proved to be quite comprehensive. At the end of the six weeks full time I was ready to do my own assessments! I had to present my very first patient to my supervisor. The patient was an 8 ½ year old boy. I took a careful and extensive history from the parents, and I carefully examined of the boy, I then started present the case to my supervisor. I thought I presented it very well.

This boy was restless and unable to sit still; he showed many of signs of ADD. He had learning problems, coordination problems, as well as many sensory motor problems. In addition he did have a family history consistent with ADD. I presented the case to my supervisor. The condition was called Minimal Brain Dysfunction then. As I have said, my supervisor was a child psychiatrist; she was the wife of the Director of the Division. I felt that this boy had Minimal Brain Dysfunction. I presented the case to her, quoting all the signs and symptoms that he demonstrated and all my reasons for my diagnosis.

As I was presenting the case, the boy blurted out "Please can I go to the toilet". On his return from the toilet the signs were not as classical as they were before, but he was still active perhaps not as active as he was before he went to the toilet; but nonetheless the diagnosis was the same. He did have the family history, the personal developmental history and the signs of the Minimal Brain Dysfunction (ADHD).

I saw a child suffering from childhood schizophrenia. When I asked the parents to come in for interview, the paternal grandparents came to the interview as well. Apparently they also lived in the family home. During the interview I picked up a few words when they were talking to the child's mother. The grandparents told the daughter in-law that it was her fault that the child was the way he was. They did tell her in Spanish as I do speak Italian so I picked up a few words that are similar to Italian. I picked up the word Diablo, which sounded like the devil. To their surprise I asked how they felt the devil was involved. They blurted out "that she knew why!" I did explain to the mother that these things happen and they are not explained by the devil causing them. I checked into the family history one of the father's 2nd cousins was in an institution and suffering from paranoid schizophrenia! A mother's worry and anguish because she often feels responsible of her child's problem is bad enough without people accusing her of causing the child's problem, and it is certainly worse when it is for an unfounded reason.

When we started the job with Child guidance; I asked my supervisor if she knew of a kindergarten that we could start our 4 year old daughter at. She told me of the Paddington kindergarten, that they did not have a waiting list. However it did have a large number of indigenous children. We did not mind, as we had been to New Guinea so we did start her there. I suffered with Dengue fever when I was in New Guinea; as a result I get very dizzy with any URTI (upper respiratory tract infection). I was lying in bed with a cold dying, dying as my wife says; when my 4 year old daughter jumped on my bed. She had been teaching her 3 year old brother this new word she has just learnt a kindy. You can just imagine what the word was, it starts with an f and ends with a k. Evelyn heard her and told her it was not a good word but my daughter insisted that she had heard it used often at kindy, and it was a good word. Evelyn then told her to go and tell me the word. I hate movements when I am sick, so when my daughter jumped on the bed it was bad enough but when she told me to get fucked I just sat bolt upright. I did not have to say anything, because she hopped off the bed and went back to the kitchen and said to Evelyn "it is not a good word is it!"

We did settle in Brisbane, we lived for 2 years in Everton Park (a Brisbane Suburb). It was reasonably close to Wilson Youth Hospital where I spent some time. My training involved a stint at the Wilson Youth Hospital. It was in no way a hospital. It was actually a detention center for youths that had offended against the law. At that time there was a law called "in need of care and control by the Department of Children Services." That Department now has a new name; I believe it is now called The Department of Aboriginal Affairs and Family services.

Any way Wilson Youth Hospital was then a cooperative joint institution, between the Department of Children Services, Corrective services and our Department; the Department of Child Guidance, a Division of the Heath Department.

Our Department was involved in providing psychological help to the wayward youths. One day, I was ready to go home at the end of my shift. I discovered that I had locked keys in my car, the old Fiat. I tried to get into the car with no joy. I had been trying for at least ½ an hour, so finally I returned inside and I got one of the youths in the place to come with me to get me into the car. He was in Wilson for the illegal use of motor vehicles. When he came with me to the car, he reached down between the driver side window and the car's panels with a lever and opened the car driver's door in a few seconds. I got the car keys, locked the car and took him back to the facility. Essential skills for any child to have! I believe that today's cars are not that easy to break into.

On another day; a white Russian therapist who was renowned to be good as a therapists; was employed by our Department and working with a group of youths. He had in his group a big indigenous lad who was an elective mute. By that, is meant that he choose not to speak to anyone. The therapist was getting his group to come up with "uck words"; the group was cooperating well so he decided to directly involve the lad with elective mutism. At first he got no response, so he persisted. The lad got annoyed with him and he eventually replied "fuck". He seized on the lad's response, and said "good" and wrote it on the black board. Just as he wrote it on the black board; the manager from the Corrective Services Department entered his room with a group of ministers; he was showing them his great facility. You should have seen their faces; they were thinking what are these lads being taught? He did explain to the ministers what had happened. Everybody did understand then and the therapist was congratulated for breaking through to this lad.

When my children started school we met a lovely family that we still keep in contact with.

Her children and my daughter went to the same school and in fact were in the same class. Soon after the children started school she invited my children to her child birthday party. We took our children over to her house and as it was a child's party we left. I thought this would be a good afternoon to be amorous to my wife. As we had not been long in Brisbane I did not know the area well yet I decide to drive about and find a lovely parking place. I found such a lovely garden; the lawns were pristine and the flowers in full bloom. I drove in and excitedly parked the car and started being amorous with my wife. Just then we heard a loud snore from the back. Unbeknown to us; our youngest child then; had crawled back into the back of our station wagon and had gone to sleep. It did not end there; as he snored I looked around more. I then realized that I had driven into and parked in a crematorium's garden (the Albany Creek Crematorium). No wonder the garden was so well kept! That definitely put an end to my plans. It has been a very funny incidence to recount now' but it was not funny at the time!

When I had completed my training, I was appointed as the Medical Officer in charge of Redcliffe Child Guidance Clinic. It was about that time that we started to live at Kallangur not far from Redcliffe.

As soon as I got to the Redcliffe clinic I decided that I would have to go to the schools in the area. As the saying goes if Mohamed could not go to the mountain then the mountain would have to go to Mohamed! Children get to spend a lot of time at school, so I decided to go to the schools in my area. Some parents are too involved earning an income to attend to their children's' needs so the teachers have so much influence on their pupils. The first school I made an appointment with was Scarbourgh State School. I made an appointment to and talk to the headmaster and the teachers. The morning of the appointment I had to sit on the toilet many times. I realized what the stress would be! I would be talking with a headmaster! I did not realize how uptight my earlier experience with the headmaster at my secondary school had left me.

I went to the school at morning tea time so that many of the teachers did come to listen to what I had to say. After all, I was the" expert" on this problem of Minimal Brain Dysfunction- as it was still called then.

I was surprised that teachers did not know much about it then even thought it was common enough and teachers had to deal with children with the "disorder" regularly. Many of the teachers were very interested in what I did have to say about the management of these children. When I finished with my talk the headmaster told his teachers "you have heard all this bullshit now go back to your class and teach your pupils!"

At the time those comments hit me like a ton of bricks. However it turned out that that was the headmaster's way of speaking. He happened to be one of the best headmasters and he tried very hard to help kids with these problems. He would often call upon me to help with advice.

Redcliffe happened to have a Bush Children's home. Children from Queensland towns without medical services were brought to these facilities to have their problems treated. There was a large number that has learning problems. The school, that I mentioned, set up a special class at his school to help the children from the Bush Children's Home with learning problems; he got a special teacher with the special skills to teach these children.

I continued with at department at the Redcliffe clinic, visiting Toowoomba clinic and later the Maroochydore clinic, (once a week).

The clinic at Redcliffe was small. The receptionist desk was crowded. As the medical officer in charge I requested the Department of Q build to come out and place some shelves on the wall next to the receptionist's desk, so that she did have more room on her desk. After waiting many months, I decided that it would be a simple matter to complete the job myself. I went to a hardware store and bought the materials and I returned to the clinic. I had the shelves fixed and in a few minutes. It so happened that that the same afternoon a carpenter from Q build arrived to attach the shelves. He found the shelves already there, so he wanted to know who had put them up. Apparently I had crossed the line of job demarcation. I was likely to cause a strike so I did tell a white lie, that "I did not know who had put them up", perhaps it was a carpenter from Q build that has come and fixed the shelves but had not written up the notes of his attendance. He accepted the possibility that a carpenter from his department had installed the selves and nothing more was heard of the incident.

My duties as the Officer in Charge of the Redcliffe clinic included several community responsibilities. I often went to kindy mothers' groups to educate them on the condition that at that time was known as Minimal Brain Dysfunction.

You can just imagine my embarrassment when the president of the mother's group called me on my mobile to ask if I was far away, I did not turn up to a prearranged meeting with a group of kindy mothers; the group had been waiting for my arrival for some 20 minutes. I was at a drive in theatre with my family. The drive in was a considerable distance from the kindy that I was supposed to be at, so the group under stood my error and just rescheduled the meeting. I only ever forgot that once and never again. Remember those early mobile telephones, they were big, I called mine the brick. Now a day they fit in your pocket.

As Professor Feingold was coming to Australia, I was asked to get a number of suitable patients that responded to the Feingold diet to present to him; he would visit us at Child Guidance headquarters. He was the the first to have described food sensitive's that was a major cause of ADHD. I was very disappointed with any diet to treat (ADHD). There are many books written about diets for ADHD but, in my opinion, they are all ineffective. The National health and Medical Research Council of Australia (NHMRC) many years ago published a paper stating that after reviewing that information from a big United States Study they could not find any evidence to support that diets affected ADHD. Although many volumes are written about the various diets they are all wishful thinking. I will discuss this topic in detail later in this book.

I was very involved with the Foster Parents association so I would see many children in foster care. The children in foster care had many emotional and behaviour problems. I did see many children and their foster parents' in my practice I was also involved with the group "Fathers caring for Kids". I will elaborate many of the fathers' opinions later in the book. I presented the first lecture of ten series 10 lectures. My topic was that of the role of fathers as a role model. I started when the group first started and I continue with the group until it ended. I would accept their referrals in the practice in Kallangur even though my waiting list was closed for new patients.

I was part of a group that wanted to change school entry. In Queensland children could start school by the time that they were 5; provided they turned 5 by the 1st of March in that year. They did not start school till March so in my opinion these children were too young to start school. When children are not yet five, the difference in maturity is considerable. The difference of 1 year may not seem much but to a five year old one year can mean 20% of their maturity when compared to the children that are 6 soon after they start school.

I did a little study at the schools in my area, the children with their birthdays until December, January, February and March (that they turn 6 in the following year) compared to the older children that forms two thirds of the numbers of children at school. I found that the one third of the younger children; have over two thirds of the problems purely resulting from maturity. The ones that manage to cope with primary school because they are bright; even though they are less mature usually end up having problems in High School.

My children chose to repeat grade 11, one is born in January and ones birthday is in December. They are both quite bright, so we started them early at school before I realized the problems that they end up having. If they have learning problems; starting them early only complicates their problems further. The group finally got a meeting with a school inspector. We presented that the children in

Victoria do not have grades in the first 3 years, the children progress according to their personal progress, children in Tasmania have two school entries and Russian children don't start school till they turn 8. I also presented my findings of my small research. After hearing us out he told us "but our Queensland children are brighter" we had to wait till he retired before the age of school entry was changed. I do believe that the age of school entry is being put forward even more now. Are we pushing our children too early? Is our society too education obsessed?

During the time I was at Redcliffe an Office of Children Services was opened in Redcliffe. At the opening ceremony, the director of Children Services said "we would not need such a Department if some parents were more responsible". At the time I did wonder if he was being fare to the parents that were faced with dealing and managing children that have problems. On the other hand he was partly correct that some parents are irresponsible with their children.

I did some consulting and visited with the Catholic family group homes at Nudgee; they were the St Vincent's family group homes. I also consulted with and visited the Uniting Church children's homes at Nundah and the family group homes at Toombool some run by St Vincent's and some by the Uniting Church. There were several also some Family Group homes in the different suburb.

I did consult and visited with one facility that provided emergency accommodation with social workers support. It was run by the Uniting church. I gave advice to the social workers with the many problems that the resident's children presented with. I continued with that organization even after I left the Department, it was a great help to community.

I was on the "Boy's Town" committee.

I attended several meetings for abused children that I looked after.

I attended. I took part in some community immunization campaigns; I did all those community services as well as my as my clinical duties. I do keep on saying I did these things not because I am up myself, but because I want to emphasize how busy I was and how the clinic and I contributed to the local community

The Redcliffe clinic has a team comprising of a psychologist, a social worker that was often asked to do home visits, and of course there were office workers.

Sometimes a specialist child psychiatrist would visit to advise me with difficult problems that I was dealing with.

While I was at the Redcliffe Clinic of the Department of Child Guidance I started to do the first part of the DPM (Diploma of Psychological Medicine), however the distance from Redcliffe to Brisbane; and even worse to St Lucia University; meant that I was often late for lectures. I did persist for 2 years before I did give up the course.

I felt strongly that the fathers should be involved with the management of all children but especially with children that had problems and they therefore required even more help.

It was usually the child's mother that brought the child for the assessment. Occasionally both mother and father attended the appointment. If only the child's mother attended the appointment; she had relate to the child's father's the management advice I had given her. Sometimes the advice was not imparted properly or interpreted correctly and sometimes the father's denied that the problem did exist.

I started to run an evening clinic so that fathers could hear for themselves the management advice. I figured that fathers often, were unable to attend appointments during normal working hours because most fathers were working. The evening clinic became very popular so I often worked late.

Children with learning problems, Aspergius Syndrome and behaviour problems, obviously, have to be taught in schools, so I often had to communicate with the Special unit of the Education Department with the same name as ours "Child Guidance", school principals or special education personnel. I often visited and attended meetings at the school for my patients.

I do differ, in my opinion, (from colleagues), because I do believe that ADHD can be diagnosed before the child is 6 years old. Often mothers' tell me that their child was different right from babyhood.

I do however agree that medication is rarely needed in a child that young.

I started a support and management group for the parents' and the young children suspected to develop ADHD, I obtained the help of a developmental physiotherapist; she is now the head of the physiotherapy Department at the University of Queensland. She ensured that the exercises that we developed were appropriate for the children that needed certain stimulations. Management during a child's maturation period does avoid further problems down the line.

We would meet on one afternoon a week, at one of parent's place. Several of the grade 12 pupil; doing their community service; from the local Secondary High Catholic School would come along as helpers for the activities. The grade 12 volunteer would help the children and ensure they would not hurt themselves; they also helped to sort out any disagreements that the children had. Children with ADD are often impulsive and sometimes feisty. We organized an obstacle course. The course started with easy obstacles for the children; then as the children improved we challenged them more. We started with a number of different sized cardboard boxes that the children had to crawl through then they had walk along a long wooden beam; it was a 3x2 20 feet long plank; it could be inclined up or down; it was inclined further as the child got better at that part of the obstacles course; The helpers would alter the beam incline as it was necessary and as they were directed by the developmental physiotherapist (for a particular child). The helpers would initially help the children that were less coordinated children across the beams. The children's' balance is also helped by walking along the beams. We would start with the wide side first, it would then be altered to the narrow side. Again the volunteers would ensure that the kids did not hurt themselves.

Some parents had a trampoline; these were very useful so they were included in the obstacle course. The child would bounce on the trampoline, the volunteers would issue commands like how many bounces they had to perform before the child has to stop. They would then alter the number of bounces that the children would do before they had to stop. As the child progressed; the tasks would be made more difficult. A ball would be thrown at the bouncing child and the child was asked to catch it.

A rope was use to divide the trampoline mat, the child was asked to go from one side to the other side of the mat. These exercises helped coordination problems and they also helped if they had sequencing issues.

A physical bonus resulted for those children that had breathing or chest problems.

I will emphasis that the volunteers ensured that the children did not get hurt; as the children with many of these problems are prone to have accidents.

A lot of sensory stimulation input is important for many young children with problems such as ADHD.

We ensured that the tactile sense was stimulated by lots of touching their shoulders. Many of Aspergius Syndrome children hate being touched so care had to be exercised with them.

Ball games were included if they were indicated for a particular child. The ball sizes varied according to the child's competence.

A wide skate like board was constructed by some fathers that were handy. The board was 15 inches by 20 inches, on the underside ball castor are attached; these were placed 2" inches from the front about 8" inches apart. The back the castors are attached to the board some 10 inches apart and 3 inches from the edge. Some fathers even padded the boards to make them even more comfortable for their child.

The child lies on their stomach and scoots along manoeuvring the board along a predetermined pathway. As the children got better with these board's the castors are moved closer to each other thus making harder to balance and manoeuvre the boards. These boards are especially useful for the children that did not go through a crawling stage.

It is very important to make the stimulation exercises fun.

The children's parents enjoyed watching the children doing their exercises. They talked and shared their experiences with each other; it helped them to realize that there were other parents that faced similar problems with their children.

We did see the improvements in the children; with their co-ordination, their concentration, their sensory inputs, their negativity, their impulsivity, etc., and a reduction of their distractibility.

A school in Western Australia did a research project with ADD children of school age. They gave the children one session of some 30 minutes; of trampoline exercises per day; they found that the children's concentration and school results improved, purely because of this intervention. Unfortunately the research was only done for a short time (6 weeks) and with a small group. It could have been just the novelty factor. I would think that the results of a properly conducted trial with a large group would be far more conclusive showing the relationship between controlled exercise and behavioural improvements.

I was invited by the principals to conduct seminars with their teachers. I presented a lecture to the National conference of the Guidance Officers of the Education Department.

I presented a paper to the National conference of Child Psychiatrists. After the conference one of the delegates requested a copy of the model that I developed and presented at the conference. I will present that model later.

I lectured a group of army fathers about children with problem; I was quite surprise how common children that had problems were; or was it because the fathers that had children with problem attended my sessions?

While I was with Child guidance we did move to Kallangur when I started at Redcliffe.

When we were about to move my 5 year old boy told the headmistress, that would bring him home, if he could stay with her as he did not want to go to the house in Kallangur. I will describe that house later and you will understand why he did not want to go there.

I was with the Queensland Health, the Department of Child Guidance, for almost 10 years. I did have to leave it because the wages at that stage were insufficient for my growing families' needs. The wages seem to have caught up since.

Being cautious and ensuring I had an income, I initially continued to work with the Health Department, in the Division of Child Guidance' in the mornings and then in the afternoon; I started in a private general practice in Caboolture. That did work out well so I eventually left the Queensland Health Department. My particular interest in mental health and behaviour problems especially that of children, soon spread by word of mouth.

Soon the practice got a loading of children with such problems. I was invited by a parents' group to talk to them about the problems that children present including normal development and then to go on with things like ADHD and Aspergius syndrome. The interest in the parents' group was so intense that I designed six week course. I was pleasantly impressed because nearly everybody in that group attended almost every lecture of the course.

The time I spent in Caboolture was so enjoyable; the patients and towns' people were very friendly and welcoming. Caboolture was basically farming and a rural country town back then. Our practice had a cooperative arrangement with the other general practices in the town so were able to work one week end and one night in four for the out of hour's calls. I will now describe the house that we bought in Kallangur. We bought such a rundown house because it was all we could afford at time and we did need the space. It was a very large house with 6 ½ acres of land. It was 2 stories at the front and three stories at the back. It was very dilapidated and un kept on the inside and in need of renovation. There were no working door locks in the house when we first moved in. I was unable to get the day off on the day we were to move in so we got a removalist, with a the very large removal van; that semi trailer was not even enough;

so Evelyn helped to move in with our (fully loaded) station wagon. She had all the children's' toys and bikes.

I did get the following day off. So on the first morning we took possession of the property. I thought I would start to clean the house up while Evelyn was preparing breakfast for all of us. I first decided to hose down the laundry and the work shop. These rooms were at the back on the lowest level. When I went down stairs to the laundry; I thought, how good is it that that these rooms had tar paper on the floor; I started to hose the floor to clean them; just then my wife called me up for breakfast, so a opened the doors to the yard, in the hope that the floors would dry; I went up to the kitchen to have breakfast. As I started to eat breakfast; the smell coming up the stair was dreadful. I realized then that what I thought was tar paper was actually ground in sheep and goats' faeces; as the sun shone on the wet faeces the smell it generated then wafted up the stair case. After quickly eating breakfast I looked at the state of the kitchen cupboards. They were rotten because the water from the sink was not correctly connected to the drainage system so the water and only drained into the cupboards. I pulled them all out and then went to purchase some temporary cupboards. We also ended up having to get a second hand stove because only one element worked on the old stove. Thank goodness to the trading post!

All the rooms needed painting. One of the rooms was painted black. When I started to paint that room white I realized why it had been painted black! As I painted it white all the terrible swear words and graffiti appeared.

I removed two trailer loads of empty cans from the ceiling cavity. The front yard had been nicely terraced in its day however neglect had taken its toll. Is it any wonder why my young son and daughter wanted to stay with the lady that gave them a lift from school! I had to rebuild the cattle crush and renovate the sheds that cattle could use to stay out the weather. The builder next door; that became a great friend, laughed at me when I was renovating a shed. Not being a builder, I did not know that the wide part of a beam is placed on its side to prevent the beam bowing; so I did use it the wrong way, any way it was ok because I was using old well seasoned timber and it did end up only bowing slightly.

I made another mistake; I bought a white carpet for the front lounge before the front yard had been done, it was virtually impossible to clean it.

The large house consisted of two bathrooms, two toilets, five large bedrooms, an office, two verandas, a storage area under the house; I have said it had a laundry and workshop at the back,

At one stage, we had to get a roofer (plumber) to fix a leak that we had in the roof; the roof of the house was far to high for me to get up on the roof to try and fix; so I got a plumber to fix the leak on the high roof. When the plumber got on the roof my young son took his ladder away and laughed at him when he came back to come down; my young son was a little devilish; but he did return the ladder later.

We had some car wrecks in the yard one was of a Chevrolet Belair that I or one of my children were going to restore We never did get round to it however.

One of my sons brought a Staffordshire bull terrier; that his previous owner was going to shoot as the dog was not aggressive enough for hunting. My wife was full of objections (initially) to him having the dog at our place.

One day my wife was in the kitchen; the dog came up to her and then kept running to the other side of the house and back to her. So she decided to see what was wrong. When she went to see why the dog kept on coming and pushing her and then running to the other side of the house and then back to her,

She saw two men that had a car trailer on the side of the road and the side gate opened. She took the growling dog by the collar and asked the men what they wanted; they saw the dog snarling at them and they quickly said we don't want anything and we were just leaving; she told them to "shut the gate as they left"; from then on the dog became her companion. We had that faithful dog for many years until he passed away many years later. The house took a long time to renovate; but when all the renovations were completed; it was a wonderful residence. Our children loved the place and the acreages; we lived there for many years until the development caught with our peaceful 6 & ½ acres.

In fact we had a good opportunity to purchase a child care centre in Aspley at a reasonable price; however all the children objected so much; that we could not sell the Kallangur house; that ended not go ahead with the purchase. A few weeks later that child care center was purchase for big money.

CHAPTER FOURTEEN

A s I said by this time I was, working full time in Caboolture. I believed in buying locally, so there was a Chrysler dealer in Caboolture so I went to them for my new Valiant station wagon. There was one catch, I had to wait six weeks to get the new car; the dealer said he could lend me a car till mine arrived. So I agreed before I saw the car he intended to loan me;. he loaned me a Triumph sport car while I was waiting for my new car to arrive; it was coloured a bright burgundy and it had flashes painted on both of the sides and it had a whippy aerial with a rabbits tail at the end of the aerial. So for six weeks I had to put up being police bait; although I removed the rabbit's tail at the end of the aerial I would still be pulled up often by the police-going home at night. When they pulled me up I would get out of the car; then they would look at me with the look of surprise; as if they expected a hoon to be driving a car like that! I kept on checking with the dealer as to when my car would arrive but each time they told me there had been a delay I the Adelaide factory but it was ok the car would came from South Australia soon. The car did eventually arrive; some 8 to10 weeks later.

There are several incidents worth mentioning that happened while I was living in Kallangur and practicing in Caboolture.

I was renovating the Kallangur house; so I had been painting all day when I finally got to bed at about mid night; I was quite exhausted by then; but I was still thinking that there were so many more jobs to do. I just took of my paint strewn shirt and shorts; I am by no means a tidy painter; I threw them on the floor just by the bed and crawled into bed. I was nearly asleep when I got a call from an ambulance driver; he said he needed me urgently; they were attending to an elderly lady that was having terrible trouble breathing. I got up; and I reached for the paint strewn cloths that I had dropped on the floor and put them on; not thinking how they looked. Remember that I was painting that day; I am by no means a tidy painter so they looked terrible paint marked and they stunk as well. I hoped in my car; by then the Chrysler Valiant had arrived. As you may know they can really travel fast. I went on the new highway that had just been opened. If I took that way and I sped, it would only take 10 minutes from Kallangur to Caboolture. I did set off really fast; I was probably doing 100kmh; as the matter that the ambulance had called me for was so urgent. A motor bike police man 'tried' to pull me up; I waved him on and passed him! He again tried to pull me up. I waved him on again, he then took the hint; he continued to follow me. When I got to my destination and attended to the patient. He asked the "Ambos" 'Who the hell is he?' The ambulance driver explained that I was the doctor and that they had called me urgently. Naturally the policeman was quite surprised; remember how I was dressed! He then got onto his motor cycle and left. A week later, he set up a speed camera to catch me; was he surprised when my wife was the driver that came out of the Valiant! She was coming to pick me up driving our car. She had just told my son that she had to slow down because this was a favorite place for speed cameras; however, she had not slowed down enough; she was just travelling just above the speed limit. He did book her and gave her a ticket for the speeding. I was an assistant by now; when the police man that had tried to pull me up on the new highway; came to the practice to consult us about his medical problems. You should have seen his face when he walked into my room and saw me. Fun aside the poor police do see some dreadful things working on the highways. I will not disclose the details of why he was so stressed. Another very funny incident happened back then. Before the present medicare was established; the federal police would investigate possible fraud. A very pedantic psychiatric patient of mine was selected to investigate my claims. Two federal police went to his housing commission place to insure that my claims were genuine. He invited then in then he locked the door behind them and he would not let them out until he had painstakingly showed them all the claim forms for consolations he had seen me for the past years; believe me there were many! They were there for several hours; they were very relieved when he eventually allowed them to leave the unit! My profile was always causing Medicare to investigate me; as it was so different from other general practitioners. After that incident, Medicare called me to ask why my profile was so different; when after I explained what my practice involved they thanked me that I was saving them a lot of money by doing what I was doing. They said that they would ring me before any investigation was to take place and that I should warn them not to hassle some of my psychiatric patients. As far as I know I have never been investigated since that incident.

We built a new surgery in association with another medical group in the town; the facilities were so good; because they were designed to our specifications; they were like an emergency department of a hospital. We included a basic x-ray facility. My consulting room included an outside verandah which doubled as a play area for the children I would see for therapy sessions. When it was completed we moved into the new clinic with the other group.

Unfortunately we had all the teething problems of a new cooperative practice. The wives did not get with each other, so we employed several receptionists. Most of my appointment should have been booked in of an hour; however the receptionists often booked the appointments in for only a fifteen minute; I would see so many children and their parents; so I often ran very late. The cost of our overheads escalated to the point that we were working to pay wages and expenses. I did persist because the facilities were great but the group practice did not work out well for me.

While I was still there; I was on call one weekend, when an ambulance brought me a patient. The patient was having anaphylactic reaction so the ambulance driver thought he could get my patient to me sooner than he could get him to Redcliffe Hospital emergency department.

When the ambulance arrived the patient was unconscious; he was sweating profusely, he was in shock; he could not breathe and he was nearly moribund. He was dying in front of my eyes. I tried to find a vein to insert an intravenous drip but I could not find a vein because of his collapse and very low blood pressure. I was shaking because I feared that I could loose him at any time. I did manage to insert a central venous line; I was so grateful to my post graduate training at Geelong Hospital because they had taught me to how to insert central venous line. The ambulance trolley had already been inclined with his head down and he was already on oxygen. I had given him intramuscular adrenalin however his circulation was so poor initially that he absorbed the intramuscular medication ever so slowly. As soon as the central venous line was inserted; I was able to give him the appropriate treatment- I started the intravenous fluids and cortisone thereby his circulation quickly improved.

I was so relieved when he started breathing.

I was then able to ask him what had happened. He told me that was helping his mother cleaning the prawns for their Christmas Dinner. He already knew that he was very allergic to prawns, but he did not realize how severe allergy was. He just wiped his hand across his lips. That must have been enough to get the reaction he got. He could not remember anything that happened after wiping his lips!

He did not have to go to hospital as he recovered fully just as quickly as he became sick. I am sure that some of my grey hairs are the result of that encounter! As the practice became busier an interstate doctor came to work in our practice as a locum; he showed an interest in staying with our practice. I eventually did sell my share of the practice to him; we agreed on the price. He paid up amount the amount that was my share; that it had cost me to build the clinic. He and agreed to pay the rest in installments (for the good will later and equipment).. When it came time for the other payments he refused and reneged on his original agreement. I had accepted a hand shake as our agreement. It would be difficult in court to prove the hand shake as no one else has witnesses it. So don't accept a hand shake agreement and get a written agreement. What has happened to trust?

After I sold my share of the group practice, I moved to Kallangur; as I had lived there for many years it was a natural choice. I met with the local practitioners that were in the area when I first came to set up the practice in Kallangur; I wanted to discuss the setting up a new practice in their area. I explained that I my work was with psychiatric problems and with children and their families that had problems including, behaviour problems. They responded that there was a big need for this sort of practice and that they would welcome such a practice in their area. Nowadays, it seems "old hat" to ask the local practices for their approval, before one makes the move into their area. It does seem that because of the acute shortage of practitioners, doctors just set up their practices when they want to; regardless of what other doctors that are there already think. It has led to situation in some in areas there are many doctors in city and suburbs but some small country towns they are screaming foe doctors and they seem to be unable to attract any.

In past time a doctor's practice was his superannuation (fund), however not many practitioners can sell their practices now; so with the result that many don't have superannuation in the way they used too.

I first set up in Kallangur in the now defunct Space City. That was a really good surgery; the rent was very reasonable because by the time I got there the shopping center was not doing well.

My wife and children saw 'Space City" being built, It was constructed of "Bennie" shells. Concrete was laid on large plastic balloons; wet concrete was poured on big balloons; while the concrete was still wet the balloons were inflated. When the concrete set the balloons were removed. The result was a dome structure. A shopping centre was made using several domes.

Unfortunately the shopping center was never successful, so when cracks developed in the concrete of the domes; the shopping centre was closed. I then moved to a shopping center at the front of a caravan park in Goodfellow's road. Space city was then demolished. I was at Goodfellows for several years. It suited me well; I saw many young children and although it was on a main road the building was set a long way back from the road. In front of my surgery was a lovely garden with several seats. My general practice side of things consisted of patients from infancy to (80+)old age. It was very interesting and varied. Some of children I delivered in New Guinea; moved with their parent's to Brisbane. They came to see me for their problems as well as their own children with their ailments and for their immunizations. I felt quite old when I saw the children of children that I had delivered!

The other side of the practice involved psychiatric problems; including depression, anxiety, ADHD, and many others. Some parents and foster parents that I had seen at Child Guidance sought me out and came to my practice.

Very soon I was very busy!

I will describe several of the very funny incidents that occurred while I was at Goodfellows Rd. Kallangur.

I have a well-known habit of poking out my tongue; it probably started when I was concentrating but it now happens without thinking. At that time my rooms in Goodfellows Rd, were in a shopping centre in front of a caravan park. One day a woman, a going to the Caravan park, pushing a her baby in a pram, went past my surgery; just then I was coming out of my consulting room; I do not remember what it was for; she looked at the name on the door and then looked at me and then she poked her tongue out at me (as I do). Apparently she could not accurately remember the name but she vividly remembered my habit. So she did use my habit to be sure it was the doctor she had seen me as a child many years ago.

After that day, she would often call in to recall old memories. She did bring her children to be immunized; she told her brother; that I had also treated as a child; where I was he too then came to see me. I did not see her after she moved from the caravan park.

We had a break-in at Goodfellows Rd surgery; the thieves only took my all immunization doses; at that time there was a measles outbreak and a shortage of those measles immunizations (medicines). I think they wanted them for the "black" market. '

Anyway we did call the police; the original door was plywood so they advise us to get a solid backdoor so we did. The next time we had a break in the thieves just cut round the locks in the solid back door. We called the police again; when they came and advised we get a security doors, this time! We had many louvre windows that thieves could get into the surgery if they wanted too; so I did not take their advice. Instead I spoke to some other surgeries; they told me that they just put up a sign 'that no drugs or money is kept on the premises' seems to deter thieves. At first I thought thieves probably can't read, so it probably won't work but in any case it was worth a try so I did put the sign up; that read; 'no drugs or money kept on the premises at night'. We never did have another "breakin" from that day on.

The Goodfellows Rd. shopping centre too was also closed (for rebuilding). So we had to move again. I, again found rooms at a reasonable rental, and although they were on the main road; again the building it is set well back off the road.

The building was originally a squash court, so it did have wooden floors. My wife who was the practice manager and all our staff appreciated the wooden floors. The floor at Goodfellows Rd was a concrete floor only covered with thin carpet. A point of interest we moved into the Anzac surgery a day before my second daughter wedding day.

We did have a truly family practice. The waiting room had a wall full of my family's pictures; the patients did seem interested in asking about the family; they enjoyed being involved in that way. The children (patients) as well saw that it was a family practice.

Evelyn referred to the patients by their name when they called for a chat, an appointment, to see how late I was, or to ask about some problem; they very much appreciated that she recognized them and that they were not just a number to us. So much so that a patient nickname Evelyn as the dragon lady- that is really an indication of how relaxed our surgery was. Evelyn is double certificate qualified Nurse so she is a real asset with her advice. I don't have a good sense of time; in fact it is quite terrible. Evelyn tries to help, by buzzing me on the telephone, close to the end of the time of a consultation. I often concentrate on the consultation, that I don't take notice of her buzzing. The patients often tell me "Doctor your wife has buzzed you several times". They have come to accept that that is my way; they know that when it is their turn they will get their time and more. They do ring the surgery to find out how I am going for time and am I ready for their appointment. Evelyn tries to estimate how long I will be. Sometimes the patient comes when Evelyn tells them to come but I am not ready for them yet; it is a usually way past their arranged appointment time. Luckily there is a good coffee shop close by and most patients do practice patience. I really don't keep an eye on the clock as I do consider that it is of the utmost importance, to carefully hear a patient out, even if it means going overtime. In order to save valuable time, when I was already late; I often found myself writing up records of the consolation's when I got home. I do realize that it is very frustrating to many patients if I am so late for their appointment; some do elsewhere but many ended coming back.

I did have a full and overflowing waiting list and I have to work very long hours. Both for my mental health patients and the my general practice side of things

CHAPTER FIFTEEN

We have had many patients for such a long time. So when it came to retire we kept on putting retirement off.

My wife suffers with a type of inflammatory arthritis called Psoriatic arthritis'. At one stage she could not even cut her own steak; she sees this rheumatologist regularly and she has helped her enormously; so much so that she could not cut her own steak before we started seeing her; now she can cut her own steak. The Rheumatologist is generally jovial, but on this particular occasion she was deadly serious; she stared directly in my eyes and said, "you know, she (my wife) won't go on forever- so do things while you can".

So with that I had to seriously consider retiring.

I was concerned as how I could retire; especially when there is such a doctor shortage. Whom would I refer patient to?

I was totally relieved when I did discuss retiring with some of the patients that I did have for a long time. They were and were getting older; so change for them would be even harder. Almost all of the patients were very understanding and many commented "you have served us well for many years so now this is your time".

I was to retire knowing that most of my patient would be ok; so with this reassurance my wife and I decided to retire.

Usually when a doctor retires from a practice he gives his patients a good bye party. I was so moved that I will have to tell you more what happened.

We consulted our accountant, and he advised me to retire in June at the end of the financial year. When we made the decision to retire, we faced a mammoth job to clean out the surgery that we had been at for some sixteen years. Luckily, a receptionist that had worked for us when she was only sixteen had come back to work with us part time. She really helped us enormously to move out. If it was not for her great help we would have of never moved out in time. Her husband also helped us. Just by the way they do have five young children. Another patient sent his father and he came with their removal truck and two men to take things that we did not need to the dump. They only accepted a carton of beer for their help.

The part time receptionist that I talked about previously; with another patient organized a party for us. They contacted the local state government member; who organized and sent out the invitation to past and present patients; she also was able to get a city council hall rent free for the evening; she also actually came and helped at the party.

At the party, so many people had come to the party many of the cars had to park on the street as the large car park was full. I estimated that there were some two hundred people at any one time; some went; while others arrived.

My wife and I were so moved to see past patients that we had not seen for a long time. We were moved so much to think that they had appreciated us so much that they had made the effort to attend. Most of the current patients were very well represented. We received so many apologies from patients that wished that they could come, but because of various reasons, they could not be present.

It was so heartening to see a young patient that we had seen previously been unable to come to a venue with a large crowd because of their anxiety, making a great effort to be there.

The catering had been organized by several of my other patients, so there was all manner of foods and plenty of it.

One patient had got a photograph us when we were in New Guinea and had it blown up and framed for us. In that picture we both looked so young; Evelyn was wearing a miniskirt and had ponytails; we were carrying our second child in the photo graph. All our children had made the effort to be there; they all had a hearty laugh at the picture and how we and the older children looked then.

When it came time for the speeches so many patient had a say; even some patients that I saw as children made a lot of effort to say a few words.

They directed their words to me and to Evelyn saying that they were grateful of the efforts that we had both made to get them through their difficult years.

A representative of the Morton Bay City Council presented us with many gifts from the Redcliffe council. He presented me with a framed certificate thanking me for the long service to the community and wishing me a happy retirement. This certificate was from the local Member of the Australian Government, The Honorable Peter Dutton. I did not know that he even knew of me!

Although we were in the Pine Rivers area the Major of Pine Rivers could not come so she sent her apologies.

When it came our turn to make a speech, we were very emotional. We told them that we would always miss our patients that had become our good friends and that we would never forget them, but "we would not miss the paper work that was involved in keeping the practice going".

The organizing pair was given many donations from very willing patients, both present and past. With the donations with that they received the organizers got us many presents. Several of the patients also wanted to give us their own personal gifts.

It was a very emotional and moving night; we will always treasure the memory of that night and all the good wishes that all the patients gave us.

At one time I attended a seminar on the subject of personal development; it was help on the Sunshine Coast at the Twin Waters Resort. I do remember being asked what my wish for life is. I said that I would like think that on my death bed I look back on my life and think it was worth having been here.

I could look back and think that the purpose of my life was fulfilled; I had made a substantial difference to peoples' lives.

The speeches by so many people with problems including those with anxiety disorders confirmed that I had made a positive difference to them.

Not too many people have the opportunity; while they are still alive; to have the recognition we had on that night.

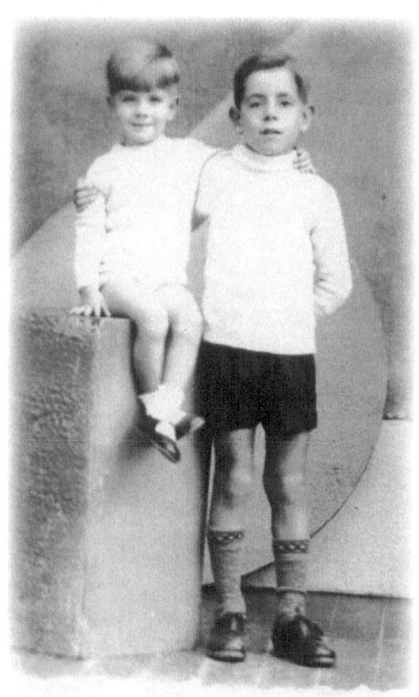

Photo of me (on left) and my middle brother
(unfortunately now deceased). I was about 3 or 4

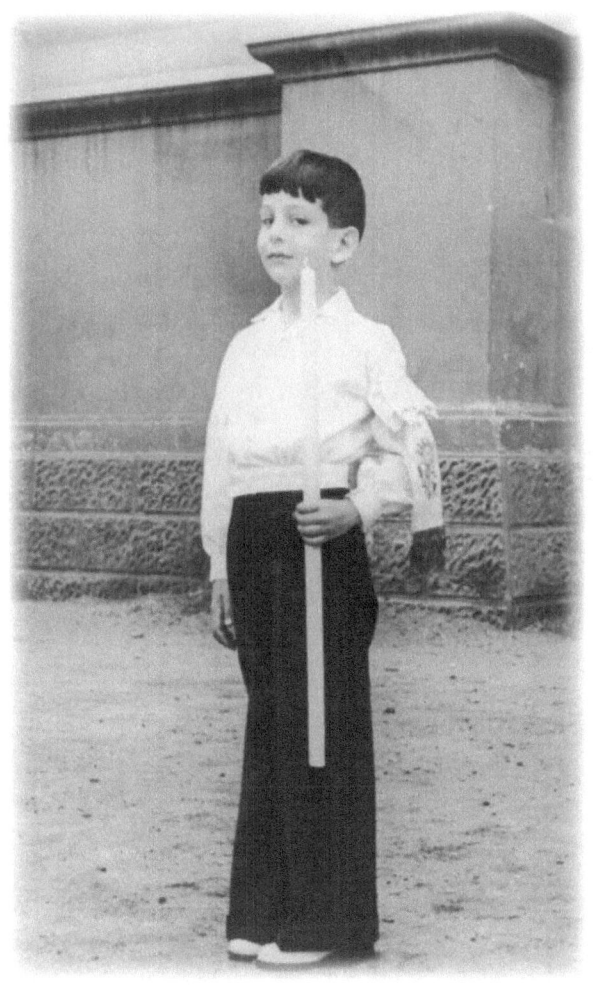

Me at age 7 or 8. Confirmation photo

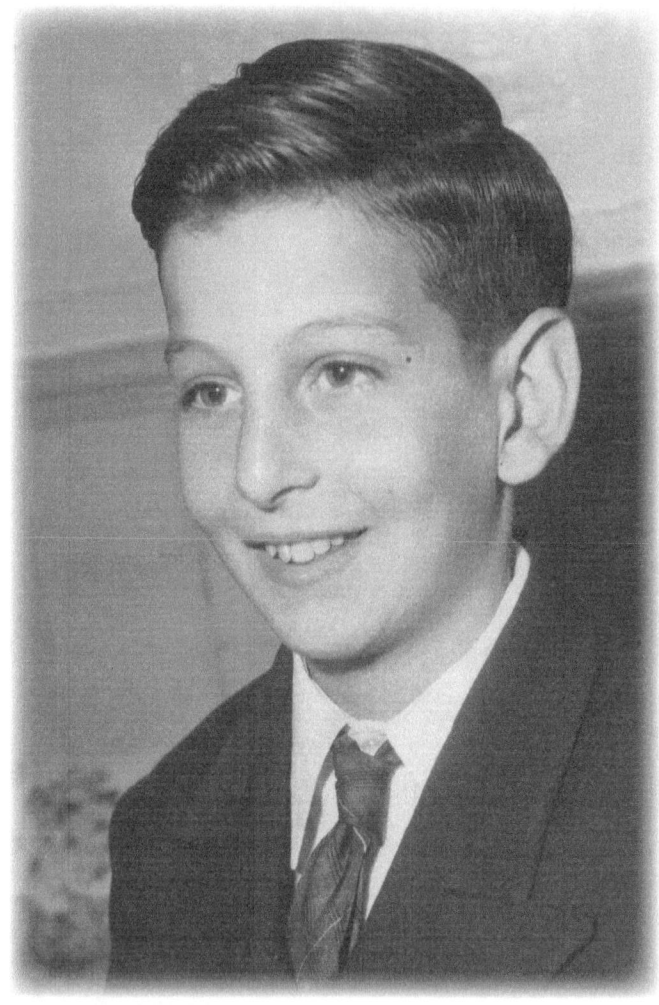

In school uniform soon after arriving in Australia

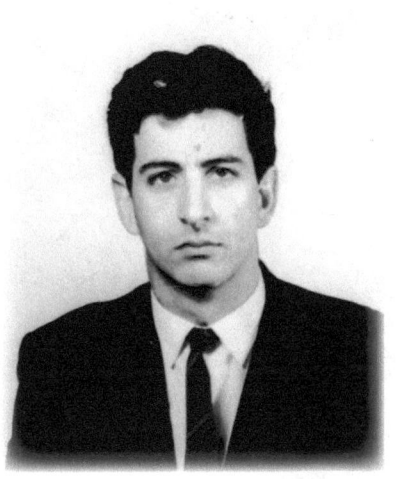

Dr. Robert Garsia, MBBS. Graduation day,
Melbourne University Medical School

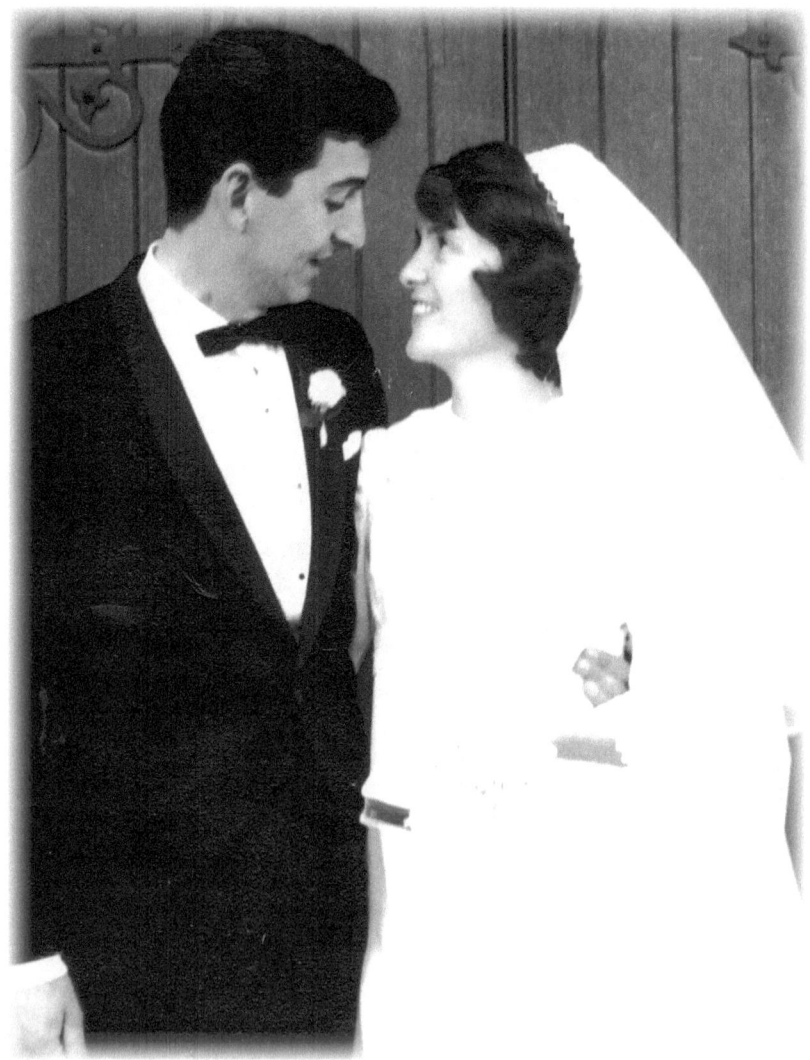

Evelyn and myself on our wedding day, May 20th, 1967

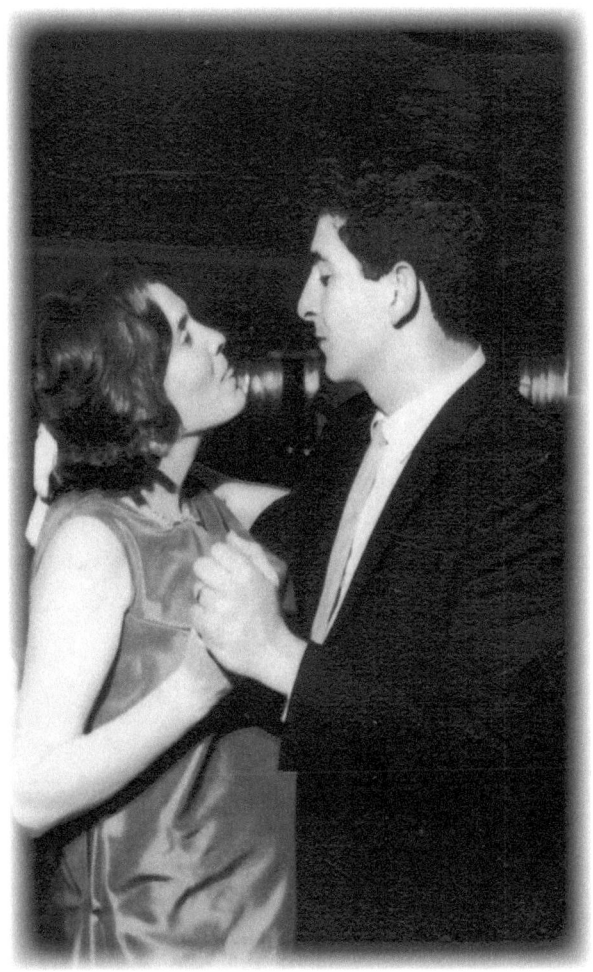

*Evelyn and I at a wedding. Evelyn was
pregnant and had made her own dress*

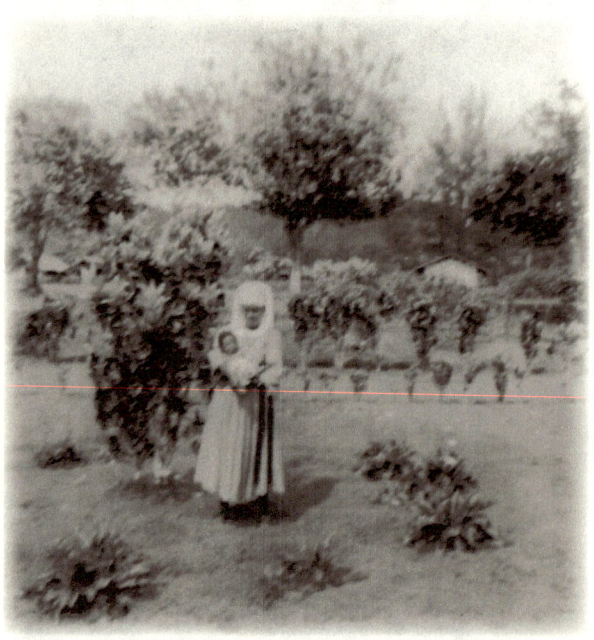

*Native nun from New Guinea
with a local infant at Vunapope mission*

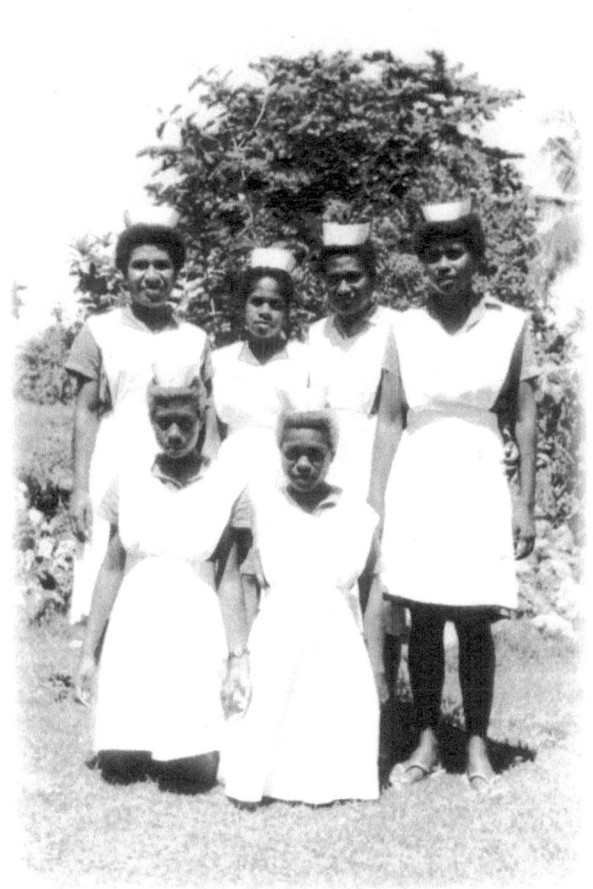

Native student nurses from the school of nursing
at Vunapope Hospital. Evelyn was one of their teachers

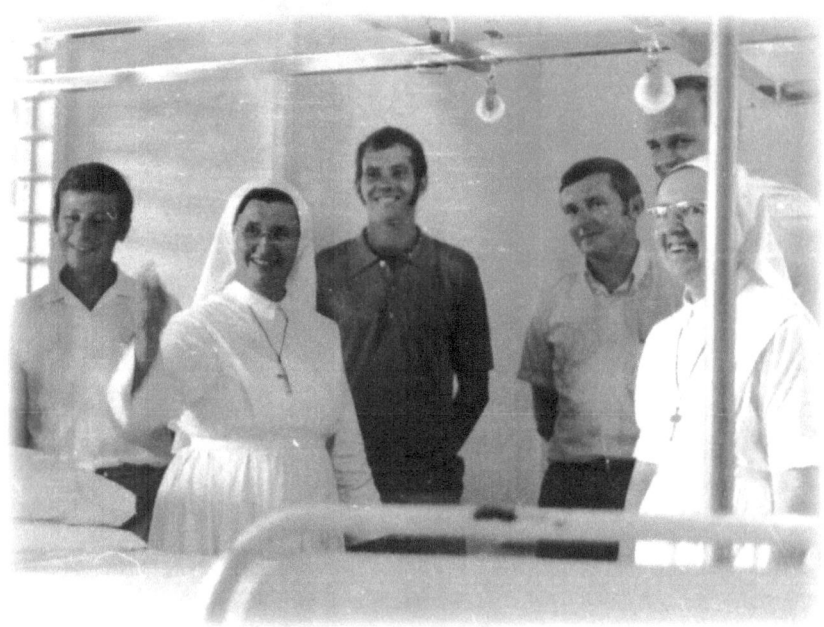

The nursing nuns gratefully accepting a donation
of an orthopaedic bed for the mission hospital.
The men were from the service club that donated the bed

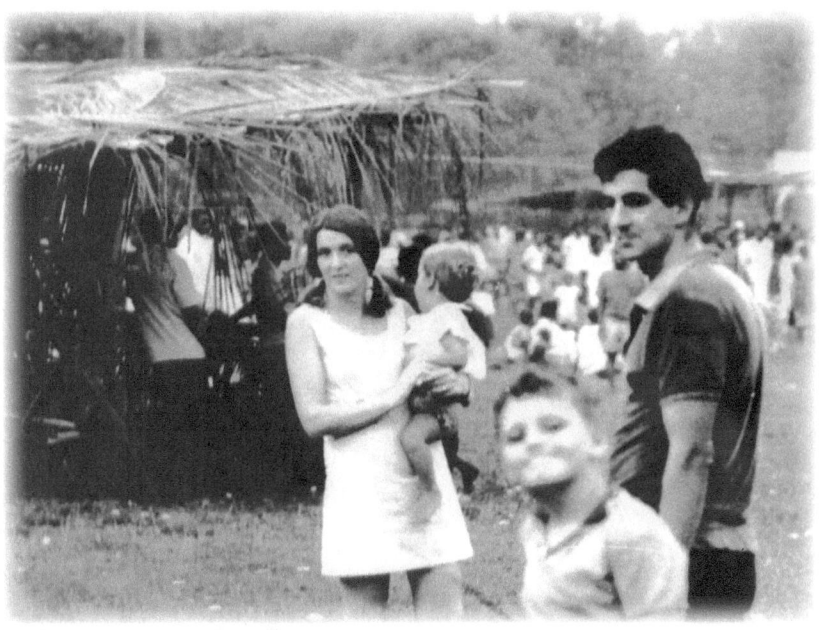

Vunapope mission near Rabaul, New Guinea in 1970. This photo was
presented to us at the retirement party that my patients gave me.
Evelyn was carrying our older boy in the photo

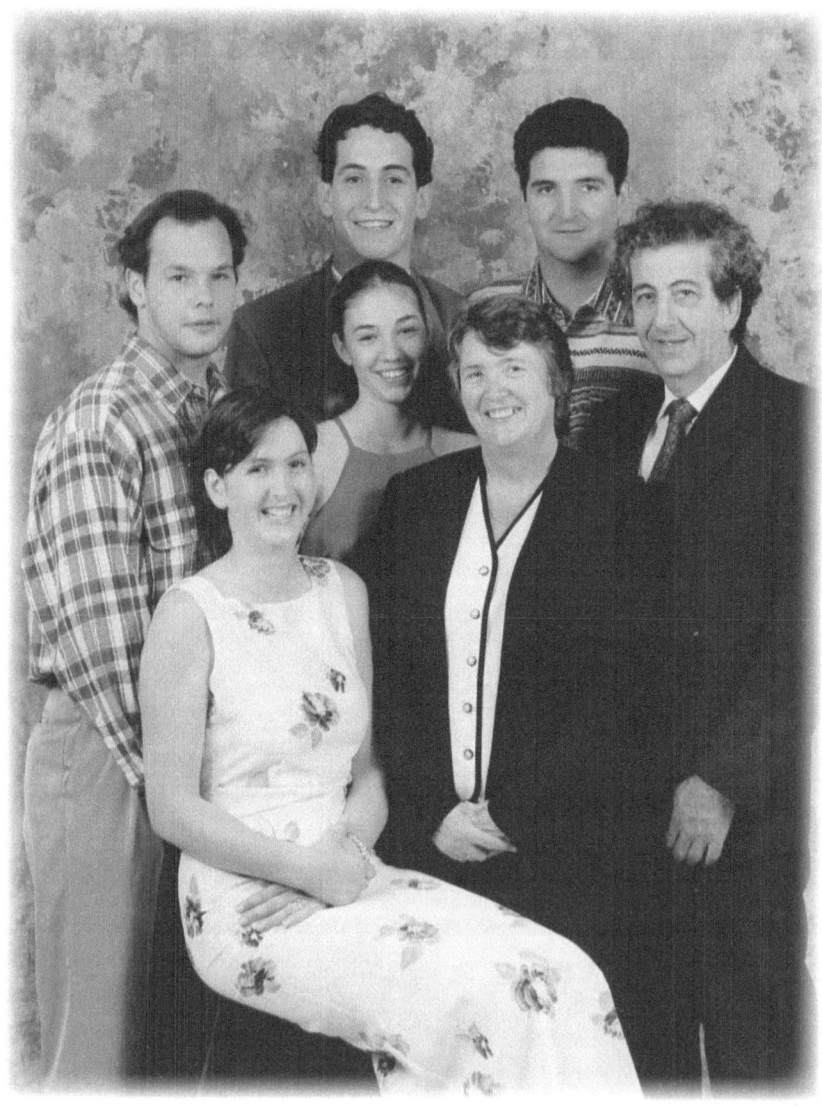

*Family portrait, unfortunately the older two children
and their spouses were unable to be present for the photo*

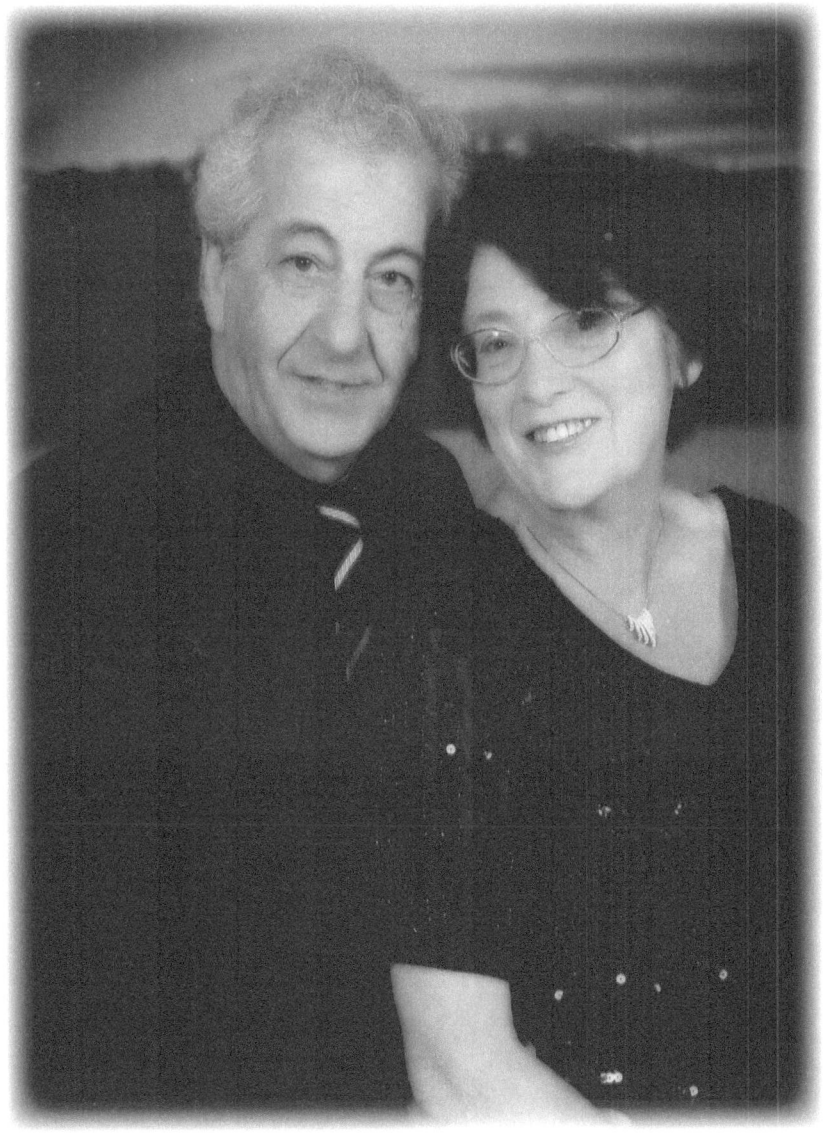

Evelyn and myself on a recent cruise

PART TWO

ADD, ADHD
AND ASPERGERS

CHAPTER SIXTEEN

———◆》·《◆———

I wanted to keep up with my medical skills (that I had learned doing my general training for the MBBS degree), so I did set up a practice with a mixture of general practice and the mental issues like ADHD, ADD Asperses syndrome, bipolar disorder, depression, anxiety, schizophrenia, sleep problems, weight control problems like anorexia and bulimia, school phobia, the list goes on and on, the diagnosis and the treatment of these conditions and the many problems that children, adolescents and adults have.

I learnt a lot first hand; dealing with these problems from the patient's themselves; of what they were going through and what they had to deal with. I did find that often psychiatric problems were not dealt with properly; by that I mean that many only received 'band aid' treatments. The Government ended up dealing with these patients in a way that I called a revolving door facility; the patients were admitted for a short time, their immediate symptom was treated but not their underlying condition; which did require long term treatment; they were then discharged, only to re-present again with their underlying problem that were not addressed in the first place-perhaps the demand of the services and the funding only allowed for short term treatment; however it did seem a short sighted vision to repeatedly have to treat the same patient again and again. Let alone that we do know that psychiatric condition deteriorates the longer they are left untreated for their psychiatric problem.

Another major problem that I encountered was that the facilities for teenager and children were few and far in between. They were some but they were mainly in city areas. The patients that suffered with drug induces psychiatric problems were often in no man's world; the psychiatric services refused to treat patients as soon as they heard that drugs had been used. The drug services seemed put off with psychiatric symptoms and a diagnosis of such a problem. Remember that psychiatric patients are more likely to use drugs; and we do know that the longer effective treatment is delayed the psychiatric condition deteriorates The children with ADHD and all the other problems were referred to me by many agencies; such as other GPs, school Guidance Officers, school principals and teachers, remedial teachers, sporting club coaches and church ministers and so on. Some came to me directly from the concerned parents themselves. Sometimes the parents had heard about me by word of mouth or the father's group-The group was called "Fathers caring for kids".

Even though my 'books' had been closed for a long time I did accept referrals from that group ("Fathers caring for kids"). I have been a foundation presenter with that group.

My opening presentation was that of the importance a father's role as a role model- that of course is a very important topic; it was the first the first lecture/presentation/discussion of a series of ten presentations.

When the referral comes from GPs; the child has been medically screened already. However I don't take that they have been examined for granted, so I proceed and take a proper and full history, and then a full examination. It is a very interesting that ADHD or ADD is much more common in boys than girls. I do see some girls with these problems. Both sexes usually do have a family history of the same problem; although the similar behaviour by one or both parent may be have been or is present is often denied by that parent at first.

Children with ADD or ADHD etc. present with a mosaic of symptoms. All these symptoms and signs may not be present in one child, but usually there is a combination of symptoms and signs.

I will describe most of the symptoms and signs that they may present with; but do remember that they may not be all present in any one child. The hallmark symptoms of the child with ADHD are a <u>heightened activity level</u>, <u>poor concentration</u>, <u>poor concentration</u> and <u>heightened distractibility</u>. All ADHD's are hyperactive; however some don't have hyperactivity problem and are very quiet; they do have ADD. ADHD stand for Attention Deficit Hyperactivity Disorder and ADD stands for Attention Deficit Disorder. These children; without the problem of hyperactivity, are at risk of being missed, because they don't cause problems to their teachers or their class mates, but they still do suffer from many of the other problems that ADD have.

Continuing now; with the other symptoms that ADHD and ADD children may present with.

They may start with <u>speech problems</u> and then go on to have <u>learning problems</u>. Some have <u>tactile problems</u>, <u>auditory</u> and or <u>visual processing problems</u>, , <u>coordination problems</u>, some have difficulty with <u>laterality</u> (telling their left side from their right side), many have <u>memory problems</u> and many may suffer with <u>anxiety</u> and <u>social interactional difficulties</u>. That is very often seen with

Asperger's syndrome. ADD and ADHD can co-exist with Asperger's Syndrome.

Some are very <u>persistent</u> and are <u>outgoing</u>.

Lots of these children many have developed <u>secondary</u> <u>behaviour problems</u> or <u>conduct disorders.</u>

They may have <u>physical symptoms</u> like <u>vasomotor rhinitis</u>; it may-mimics allergy.

<u>Enuresis</u> (bladder control problems) and/ or bowel problems such as irritable bowel and / or constipation may be present.

<u>Appetite</u> can be variable; they can be <u>anorexic</u> or <u>bulimic</u>; they don't want to put on weight; by not eating or vomiting just after eating; because they have an abnormal body image, or they have an appetite which cannot be satisfied; sometimes it is only for certain foods, sugar for instance.

Many have <u>sleep problems</u>.

Many have <u>temper control problems</u>.

Some may be very <u>literal.</u> Many often admit to <u>misbehaviour</u> when they are asked if they did do something wrong, but they don't think to say how they were provoked.

Some are <u>emotional</u> and or are easily up set and they may be <u>labile</u>.

They are easily set up because of their reputation; they may or may not deserve; but they may have gotten the reputation themselves.

Many can be <u>easily influenced</u>; the other children know that they can get them to do things so as it is said they can make the "bullets" and let the child in question fire them.

They are often <u>loud</u>. They are the ones that the teacher hears, so the teacher believes they are the ones that are responsible for most of the things that do happen in the class room.

They often gravitate to other <u>children with similar problems</u>.

They may <u>react quickly</u> to being stirred.

They are often caught <u>fighting</u> and they are often <u>impulsive</u>.

Most schools don't allow their pupils to get into fights. They are told to go and tell the teachers if they are provoked, but not to fight, but they are to report bulling to the teachers. A lot of the time when they do go to tell some teachers often they are told not to be 'tattle tales'. In our day, children were told to stand up for themselves even if it meant that they would have to fight the child that was bulling them.

They are can be very <u>inquisitive</u> and they find it very hard to stay out of things that don't concern them. They often want to be involved in adult conversations.

It is worth repeating, that many have difficulty with sleep. They may have trouble going to sleep, they may have trouble because of waking early; they need a lot of sleep or they don't sleep enough.

I have mentioned some of the <u>eating fads</u> that are common.

They may have <u>funny tastes</u>. They may always be the sugar bowl.

They often take thing apart and forget to put them back together again.

They often have poor <u>organizational</u> ability especially when it comes to getting the things they need to get ready for school.

They are always very keen to start a new activity, such as learning a new instrument, joining a club, maybe to play a sport; or a social club. The parents always ask them to be sure that that is what they want; they are adamant that is what they want, so the parents buy the expensive gear that is needed for their chosen activity. Soon the child decides that they want to do another activity; perhaps they did hear from a friend how good this alternative activity is so they discontinue their initial choice and want something else.

As you can realize there are so very many possible combinations of behaviours that they can present with; before the correct diagnosis can be made let alone that the correct treatment is prescribed. A conduct Disorder can result from the many symptoms that untreated ADHD child has.

They are often in trouble.

Many have got a bad reputation because they have many if not all the symptoms. They may have some problems doing some things; their sibling may not have trouble doing the same things, but the teachers may be tempted to compare their achievements and their skills to their siblings. They may say your "your sibling does so much better". To make matters worse their sibling may be younger.

Is it any wonder that this often to why they often have such a <u>poor self-esteem!</u>

I do often use a 'questionnaire' to enquire about the child many behaviours.

I ask the parents to fill one each and to get the child's teacher to fill one out also.

On some occasions the parents disagree with each other about the child's attributes; sometimes the teacher's response are quite different about the child's behaviours at school. I do also compare the parent's individual answers to the; the teacher's responses as the teachers are nearly always unbiased. The parents' responses on the questioners may be different; that often suggests that one parent denies that their child of theirs could possibly have a problem; interestingly enough it is usually the parent that did have the same problem when they were young! The teacher's may see a lot more of the problems because ADHD children can be so different in different situations; it may be that at school there are more distractions because of so many other children in the class. Example of the typical ADHD and an Aspergius syndrome questionnaire are enclosed!

ADHD RATING SCALE IV – HOME VERSION
(University of Massachusetts Medical Centre-Modified)

Childs Name...Grade.......................

Date of Assessment ....

Completed By ....

Circle the number that <u>best describes</u> your child's home behaviour recently

	Never or Rarely	Sometimes	Often	Very Often
Fails to give close attention to details or makes careless mistakes in his/her work	0	1	2	3
Fidgets with hands or feet or squirms in seat	0	1	2	3
Has difficulty sustaining attention in tasks or play activities	0	1	2	3
Leaves seat in classroom or in other situations in which remaining seated is expected	0	1	2	3
Does not seem to listen when spoken to directly	0	1	2	3
Runs about or climbs excessively in situations in which it is inappropriate	0	1	2	3
Does not follow through on instructions and fails to finish work	0	1	2	3
Has difficulty playing or engaging in leisure activities quietly	0	1	2	3
Has difficulty organizing tasks and activities	0	1	2	3
Is "on the go" or acts as if "driven by a motor"	0	1	2	3
Avoids tasks (eg. Schoolwork, homework) that require mental effort	0	1	2	3
Talks excessively	0	1	2	3
Loses things necessary for tasks or activities	0	1	2	3
Blurts out answers before questions have been completed	0	1	2	3
Is easily distracted	0	1	2	3
Has difficulty awaiting turn	0	1	2	3
Is forgetful in daily activities	0	1	2	3
Interrupts or intrudes on others	0	1	2	3

ASPERGERS QUESTIONARES

Child's name _____

Age _____ Sex: M / F

Birth Order: Twin or single birth _____

Parent / Guardian _____

Parent(s) occupation _____

Address _____

_____

Phone# _____

School _____

Please read the following questions carefully, and circle the appropriate answer.

Does s/he join in playing games with others easily?
Yes
No

Does s/he come up to you spontaneously for a chat?
Yes
No

Was s/he speaking by 2 years old?
Yes
No

Does s/he enjoy sports?
Yes
No

Is it important for him/her to fit in with a peer group?
Yes
No

Does s/he appear to notice unusual details that others miss?
Yes
No

Does s/he tend to take things literally?
Yes
No

When s/he was 3 years old, did s/he spend a lot of time
pretending (e.g., play-acting being a super-hero, or holding teddy's
tea parties?
Yes
No

Does s/he like to do the same things over and overagain, in the
same way all the time?
Yes
No

Does s/he find it easy to interact with other children?
Yes
No

Can s/he keep a two-way conversation going?

Yes

No

Can s/he read appropriately for his/her age?

Yes

No

Does s/he mostly have the same interests as his/her peers?

Yes

No

Does s/he have an interest that which takes up so much time that s/he does little else?

Yes

No

Does s/he have friends, rather than just acquaintances?

Yes

No

Does s/he often bring things to show you that interest s/he?

Yes

No

Does s/he enjoy joking around?

Yes

No

Does s/he have difficulty understanding the rules for polite behaviour?

Yes

No

Does s/he have an unusual memory for details?

Yes

No

Is his/her voice unusual (e.g., overly adult, flat, or very monotonous?

Yes

No

Are people important to him/her?

Yes

No

Can s/he dress him/herself?

Yes

No

Is s/he good at turn-taking in conversation?

Yes

No

Does s/he play imaginatively with other children, and engage in role-play?

Yes

No

Does s/he do or say things that are tactless or socially inappropriate?

Yes

No

Can s/he count to 50 without leaving out any numbers?

Yes

No

Does s/he make normal eye-contact?

Yes

No

Does s/he have any unusual and repetitive movements?

Yes

No

Is his/her social behaviour very one-sided and always on his or her terms?

Yes

No

Does your child sometimes say "you" or "s/he" when s/he means to say "I"?

Yes

No

Does s/he prefer imaginative activities such as play-acting or story-telling, rather than numbers or a list of facts?

Yes

No

Does s/he sometimes lose the listener because of not explaining what s/he is talking about?

Yes

No

Can s/he ride a bicycle (even if with stabilizers)?

Yes

No

Does s/he try to impose routines on him/herself, or on others, in such a way that it causes problems?

Yes

No

Does s/he care about how s/he is perceived by the rest of the group?

Yes

No

Does s/he often turn conversations to his/her favorite subject rather than following what the other person wants to talk about?

Yes

No

Does s/he have odd or unusual phrases?

Yes

No

SPECIAL NEEDS SECTION

- Have teachers/health visitors ever expressed any concerns about his/her development?

Yes

No

If yes, please specify_____

- Has s/he ever been diagnosed with the following?

Language delay

Yes

No

Hyperactivity/Attention Deficit Disorder (ADHD)

Yes

No

Hearing or visual difficulties?

Yes

No

Autism Spectrum Condition, including Asperger syndrome?

Yes

No

A physical disability?

Yes

No

Other? (please specify

Yes

No

If yes, please specify_____

CHAPTER SEVENTEEN

———————— ◆》•《◆ ————————

Most parents present because of the behaviour problems but the main treatment is directed to the child's hyperactivity, poor attention, heightened distractibility and concentration problems; these are the problems have that resulted in the associated problems. The behaviours, these are the main concerns that the parent want to change, The management advice is directed to the poor self image and the other many problems that the child may have; like the poor retention of information (memory problems). Many of these things have happened as a result of their original problem so management advice is always necessary to try and reverse the secondary behaviour problems. These secondary problems have resulted because the period that the child was not adequately managed and treatment and for their ADHD. The fundamental of my advice was to correct the behaviours and so to improve the child's self-esteem. They need of unconditional loving, help, acceptance and encouragement. These things go a long way to help heal the poor self esteem.

Children require limits, but not control by punishment, so quite persistent patient limits are necessary.

A reward system should be set up to encourage the child to apply themselves. The University of Queensland (UQ) Psychology department originated the Positive Parenting and courses; they have gone on to develop Positive Parenting for adolescents. If after I have discussed reward based management; the parents require more information about the reward system of management (positive parenting); many schools run early intervention courses and Positive Parenting courses. Many community welfare organizations also run these courses.

Many of the parents have their own problems, they too must also be addressed. I will elaborate on the management of ADHD later. My usual approach is to read the referral letter carefully, as the referral letter is usually very helpful; however they sometimes can be useless; the referral note may not provide me with any important details but some just referral letters just introduces the child and asks to please assess this child. Most Teachers', Education officers and headmaster's referrals are often very detailed, but they too can be short or biased. In any case the parents are well aware of the child's problems. I start by asking them why the problem was referred to me—why now, "why at this time?" I get very many explanations; some say that they did not know where to get help, others say that they did consult a doctor in the past and that they had been told 'that there is nothing wrong and the child and in any way the child will grow out of it; some say they were not satisfied with that explanation; they did know that there was a problem, but they could not afford another expensive consolation. They did know that the child did have a problem. Maybe the child would grow out of it and maybe they would not but they would miss the building blocks for their further education. They gave me the example that they knew that there was something wrong with their child memory to retain information. Their child spent a lot of time learning a list of spellings with their efforts; that they were given for home work and at the end of the evening they knew all the spelling correctly. When their child by asked by the teacher to was to spell the word that they had learnt the night before; they only got very few spellings correct. Yet the very night before; they knew all the spelling perfectly. Again and again some parents said did not know where else to go because their GP told them not to worry because when he saw the child "butter did not melt in the child's mouth'. Some parent said they could not afford help!

Many parents were desperate and wanted to see what they could do to help their child. They would often just say "how do I best help my child".

There were many similar answers to my questions I have only reported the main ones to you.

In some cases the teacher or some agency insisted that they see a doctor. Sometimes the teacher even arranged for the appointment. The teachers may have heard my lectures (during teacher further education seminars– during pupil free days) and so recognized the problems and thus referred the child to me. I am happy to say that some other professional's had heard my lectures or other specialists in field and referred children; with these problems, to a child guidance clinic, a developmental unit or to me. I believe that the Child Guidance clinic, now called Child and Youth Mental Health clinics (CYMS) for short, don't accept referrals from ADHD children unless they have emotional problems too. In my opinion all children with ADHD do have to emotional problems anyway; they have poor self esteem as well as learning problems, but as soon as ADHD is mentioned, the clinics say they should be referred to the school Guidance Officer for their learning problems. ADHD children often have many more problems than just leaning problems!

I have had great difficulty finding child psychiatrists, developmental paediatricians or practitioners that bulk bill and deal with their whole problem. Thankfully I have found several professionals that will bulk bill if they are requested to; but unfortunately their waiting list to see them is long. Mind you I do know the financial difficulties and the expenses of running a practice; and that the Medicare benefits have not kept up with the cost of running a practice so bulk billing can be a strain. Most parents do consider their children as their first priority. However there are a few who would prefer to spend their income on alcohol and cigarettes.

There are a few developmental units but they are few a far between; and as well most are in the Capitol cities. The country areas are not well represented. There are public hospitals units with developmental units but they all have long waiting lists. In my opinion, treatment of these children is often delayed too long.

Luckily my overheads were kept to a minimum; my wife's wages were kept at 1995 award level and we had premises with reasonably cheap rentals. There are many paramedical personnel that offer assessment and treatments for the various problems that these children have. Many of them don't always "bulk bill". Thankfully our Division of general practice did offer to subsidize some sessions with paramedical treatment of children and adults too.

There are many alternative treatments professing to cure ADD or to help in the treatment of the "condition".

The "condition" is common enough so many people hop on the band wagon to make money. I will raise this topic again later.

Returning now to my consultations; I often write to the schools or telephone the school teachers, or sporting clubs leaders to seek further information. When I write to schools, I address my letter to the headmaster; the headmaster then passes on my enquiry to the relevant teacher; if the child has not been in too much trouble he may not know the child. The headmaster or the teacher either write back or they sometimes ask that I ring back at an appropriate time as they wish to further discuss the child's management with me. In that way I get a rounded picture of the child in various situations; not just at home! The report is occasionally quite different to the one that the parents presented. I have already said that an ADD child is different, with different levels of stimulations. A typical letter that I do send to schools is as follows;

The head of the school involves, Dear sir/madam Re child's name, grade, dob This child is attending here for assessment and treatment. I would be very interested in any comments that your or the child teacher would like to contribute to the child's assessment; I would be very interested in any comment you or the child's teacher can offer about the child's behaviours, learning problems, activity, memory and anything that you or the child's teacher would like to like to comment about; both the class room and the play ground. Yours faithfully R.V Garsia

When a school is involved; the school teachers are very cooperative, often; they are very keen to get advice as to how best teach and handle the children with problems. I have said it not only that child that their condition affect but it most likely affects the other children in the class.

Very occasionally, bias exists in their reports that I get back; this can be either way. Either; that ADD does not exist and that all that is required for the child's bad behaviour is discipline; they do really mean (punishment). Usually they are biased people and don't believe that if a child is diagnosed properly and effective treated the child will do better with the appropriate medication.

Alternatively they believe that the reason for the bad behaviours by any child is due to ADHD; at the extreme end; there are some teachers that believe all children with behavioural problems need medication before they can effectively teach them.

Teachers are representative of the general population and so they are entitled to their opinions, however, it is the children that may suffer because of their opinions. So they should be very careful when their opinion will affect others especially children.

They may refer the child, and they demand that the child be medicated A proper assessment is needed before a child is diagnosed with ADHD and such potent medication as Ritalin is carefully prescribed. Careful follow up to monitor the effect and to carefully adjust the dose is mandatory. There are so many reports on the internet of the terrible side effects of medications; in particular Ritalin. The parents, that don't know any better when they see the dramatic reports by unprofessional reporters that indicate that this treatment or that treatment works well for ADHD; usually they indicate that the treatment does not need medication; it does imply that medication is not a good treatment, or the parents consult Dr. Google on the internet; or some 'know all' friend that tells them of a treatment that has proved effective; usually it does involve a treatment without the traditional treatment with stimulants.

All of these opinions result in increasing their anxiety, and probably the delay of the effective treatment of the child. Stimulant medication is a good medication when it is properly used. Sometimes the teachers are not as tactful as they should be when they tell the parent that they believe their child has ADHD. They may be correct; however some parents are then alienated by teacher's attitude. They then use that as an excuse to refuse to accept the diagnosis. It is often that the parents knew that there was a problem but they use this as an excuse because they were against any treatment any ways. They use the opportunity to attend the appointment that was made for them however they were against any traditional treatment any way.

I have come across such parents that are against medication under any circumstance. These parents do use any excuse they can to justify refusing effective treatment for their child. They often try all sorts of alternative ineffective treatment before them, hopefully, come to accept the correct therapy. Again it is the child that misses out! As I said some parents find it very difficult to believe that the teacher report that their child is so active and does not concentrate. That is most likely because when the child is at home can do their work well. At home it is on a one to one basis, however at school there are so many distractions. The ADHD child often becomes the class clowns because the child does have an audience at school. (That they don't have at home). When, that is explained to the parents; that the distractions in a classroom can be so many. They realize what the teacher has to deal with- the behaviours and difficulties with their child's concentration, activity, distractibility and memory problems etc. which are so different in the classroom because of the many distractions in the class room. When the parents do clearly understand; the reasons for the teacher's comments and the diagnosis; most will accept the treatment; it is not only for their child's benefit but that of the whole class. The treatment must always include management advice; follow up and in some cases medication. Most parents expect and want some test to confirm the diagnosis.

It is very important to explain to such parents that the diagnosis is made on <u>clinical grounds and how and why it is made</u>. In the history of medicine the clinical diagnosis was arrived at in the first place and eventually a test was developed to confirm the clinical findings. No <u>definitive</u> test has yet been developed to definitively confirm the diagnosis of ADHD. I will speak briefly about the incidence of ADHD in different countries. It does depend on how they choose to define the problem. Some counties apparently have a low incidence of ADHD because the problem there is considered a psychosocial problem; other countries define it as an organic brain problem; I will suggest that it may be a normal variant like hair and eye colour. In any case the child's symptoms and signs are the same. Most parents are naturally protective when it involves their child so their anxiety must be explored and they need to be assured that they are making the best decision for the child. Their anxiety is often fuelled by so many reports and so many opinions about the dramatic and rare side effects of the medications that are used for the present treatment of ADHD. What do poor parents believe, who do they believe when they are confronted with exaggerated risks of medication? I empathize with to parents that I understand their concerns. They get confronted with a great amount of the misinformation that from different areas that it is difficult to make an informed decision. Parents have not had the training to assess these reports that some research reports claim that they found 'such and such'. We do some do many years of study we then have to keep up our professional standards training updates; we do have access to the "Cochran Library" to help us to assess these reports. By the was some 80 to 90% of research projects have been found to be useless; for instance a group of researchers found that power strikes cause an increase in child births- of course the parents go to bed earlier but it is not the power strike that causes the increase in child births. Parents are told of the terribly bad side effects of the stimulant medications that are used for ADHD; such as Ritalin. Often programs and the print media and the internet portray the rare negative side effect as the norm. They may also have heard from a one or several of the self-appointed so called experts; these people have an answer of everything and what to do in every situation. The parents of these children have to put up with seeing and hearing these 'opinions'. You don't go to have your car fixed by a carpenter so why do you go to a current affair and find out how to fix your child's problems?

I do get reports that the parents of ADHD children have been told 'that all the child needs is discipline; they usually means that all our child needs is a good belting'; or they are told "Just let me have the children for one week and I will fix them". Some parents may not follow the treatment if the diagnosis and the reasons for the diagnosis and the treatment are not explained fully and carefully. One must explained by stressing that close follow up measures will be put in place and that a strict adherence to the medication regime will be followed. I come across some parents that in spite of what are the efforts that are made to explain the situation still refuse to give the child medication. Very often they spend a lot of money trying many ineffective alternative treatments. Some do end up coming back after they have been disappointed trying some of the ineffective (and usually expensive) 'treatments'; some of these are in fact some form of medication. Again it is the child that misses out on their effective treatment; or their effective treatment is unnecessarily delayed. I will discuss many of these ineffective treatments later in this book. A situation still does occur when seemingly conflicting information is given to a lay person. It does happen in medical matters also. For example, a physiotherapist tells a patient one thing, the nurse tells the patient something else and finally a doctor then says something else that sounds quite different but it is the same perhaps by a different name for the same condition. In most cases, it may actually be the same advice, however to the lay person it may seem different. Complicate this further and have advice come from different fields; like a chiropractor or maybe a naturopath-the alternative medicines field; they often do use medical terms that don't quite mean the same thing, is it any wonder that the parents can end up being confused! It is interesting to listen to quiz shows on the television how many people don't have a clue when the host asks the contestants a medical question!

Perhaps, it is because of the parents' confusion does results in the poor child missing out, or at best the delaying of getting the proper and effective treatment; medication including the correct management advice.

It is essential, and a practitioner's responsibility, to make sure that the parents of a child with ADHD or any condition including Asperger's Syndrome do really understand everything that is said to them. It is very important to answer any questions that a child or the parents may have, and result to patiently make sure they understand them clearly and fully. It is of the ultimate importance that we avoid sounding arrogant; by using our jargon; or sounding as if we are judgmental; lest the child or his parents are reluctant to ask any more questions. If parents are to accept the medication, the pro and cons of the medication must be carefully explained to them and the child' especially if the child is older. The prescribing practitioner must monitor the child's progress for any possible side effects. These include checking the heart, blood pressure and their growth.

There are so many consequences of untreated ADHD (and Asperger's) etc. I will discuss a few of them. (1). It can lead to alienation by the child because they feel rejected or over controlled; sometimes one parent finds the child's problems are too difficult to deal with, so they can end up being discipline (over control) orientated or worse, rejecting that child, not just their behaviour (It is often a parent with their own problem or similar problems to the child that may deny that the child has any problem) and so they can't/don't deal with the problem. The family friends' may stop having you or the child over because of the childs' ways-more potential reason for rejection (2). Alienation to authority; they often get in trouble with authority; some it is not even their fault or they don't think so. Is it any wonder that some don't like authority (3). The child's may end up with a poor self-esteem due to their poor coordination and/or their learning problems. These often results in their poor achievements; hence their poor self image-self esteem. (4) Again they may have poor memory and again they fail to achieve to their potential. Because of their memory problems they can have poor school results in spite of their good ability and their intelligence. Again the result is more than likely a poor self esteem. (5). They may have poor co-ordination skills so some schools are very sport inclined and applauded sporting achievements; they are far from sporty so their sporty school peers reject them because of their poor performance; the school also find their achievements in sport no good. (6). If they have poor social skills (especially Asperger's syn.) They are often rejected by their peers or manipulated by them. The opposite gender may add further to this problem because children with ADHD seem so immature-again cause for further rejection and this adds further to their poor relating skills (7). I have already stated that one or other parent may reject the child because of their own problems or because of all the above reasons that their child gets poor achievement. In their frustration they may yell and make very derogatory comments or very negative comments. I sound like I am making an excuse for them but they may have their own problems too. In any case it does affect the child and the sooner it can be sorted the better it is for the child. It may mean that that parent has to get treatment for their own problem. (8) They often cause problems to their siblings; such as fighting with their sibling or being suspended so one parent has to lose some income. The sibling may them miss out on an outing that they have been looking forward to going to; the sibling misses out because of the consequences because of their suspension so again the feeling of being rejected by their siblings and the probable poor self esteem that again can result. (9) They are more prone to other mental disorders and using illegal drugs as they approach adulthood. I will discuss this further later. As you can see there are very many negative consequences to the conditions, so early effective treatment and management advice does prevent or reduce the likely hood of further problems developing. I will later discuss a property of human development that is called a critical period. Parents often accept the correct and effective treatment for their child once they understand the complexity and the many possible consequences of not treating their child's condition as early as possible. It is vital for the practitioner to follow up with the treatment; to assess the progress; to monitor for side effects; to adjust the dose of medication as the child grows; to ensure the progress goes according to plan; to ensure that the parents understand the treatment goals and ensure that they meet the parents and the patients expectation; to communicate with anybody like their teachers, their siblings and anybody that is affected by the child's condition. It is the child that suffers if we don't do our job well or the parents don't come back for follow up appointments.

CHAPTER EIGHTEEN

The parents often explain their concerns in their own words so it is essential and very important to listen to them carefully; to exactly understand what the parents' concerns are. It is for the practitioner to understand them fully and to make sure that we do comprehensively understand them. It is just as important that they fully understand us so don't use our jargon; if you do, make sure they understand it. I have already talked about some of the reasons why parent come for a consultation. I will discuss some other reasons now. Some of these reasons are as follows, usually one parent is very concerned about the child's behaviour, but the other parent is really resistant to the idea that their child has anything wrong with them. Sometimes they are not concerned, but somebody else did insist they come for this appointment. Often they have tried different alternative preparations according to some reports they have seen or heard, with little success, but they are still trying to get the result they believed they should get. They are resolved that they would not the improvements that they thought they would get; but they eventually came to try another avenue to help their child. They have heard (by word of mouth) that maybe I may be able to help; I did bulk bill so it would not cost them much to try me for help. Sometimes they have got complains about their child's behaviour by their good friends, or their 'good' friends refused to have them back with that child. Many times it was concerned teacher, a speech pathologist, an occupational therapist or a school Guidance Officer that had brought the child's to the parents' attention and asked them to make the appointment or made the appointment for the child themselves. I would always ask the child's parent to contact me before I would give them an appointment. As I have already stated, the parents did know of the problems but did not know where to go, or they had already seen their GP and then a Specialist, only to be told the child will probably grow out of it. The advice was probably correct, "that the child would eventually grow out of it" but at what is cost to the child in the meantime. It is the poor child that suffers; they have developed more problems including a poor self-esteem. The majority of parents are relieved that at last, an effective and safe treatment is available. That finally they have a practitioner does listen to them and understand their difficulties and will try and do something about it. If the referral comes under sufferance, the parents often do not follow up with subsequent appointments in spite of explaining how important the problem is. It is important to point out that the "problem" may not be totally corrected; and the treatment will help and take time to make things better, lest their expectations are not fully fulfilled and I lose the patient. Once I have explained how important it is to have the correct diagnosis so that the correct treatment can be prescribed I do start with the past history, the history of the child's problem and I then proceed with the examination. The family history is very important; interestingly one or other parent or a close relative has had similar problems to the presenting child. I will mention a few only of these problems; they include such things as, concentration difficulties, hyperactivity or hypo-activity, distractibility, laterality problems, dyslexia, learning problems, math's difficulties and many other problems. The parent involved may have genuinely or forgotten (but that is unlikely) that they did suffer with these problem; but often the grandparents remember and offer that history, that their child; now the presenting child's parent, had similar difficulties at a similar age. Genetic factors are often present. The child gets it heredity factors from his/her parents. The chromosome in the child's DNA comes one half from the mother and the other half from the father. We have 23 pairs of chromosomes and an unpaired sex chromosome which determines the person's sex amongst other characteristics. At the time of ovulation the mother's ovaries split the pairs of chromosomes into single strands (of genes). The process is called Mitosis. As a result the ovum has a single set of chromosomes. The father's testicles do the same to the sperms chromosomes, so that the males spermatozoa have a of singe stranded chromosomes. At conception the spermatozoa penetrate the ovum so the two single strands of chromosomes are joined together to form the new unique DNA of the child. The person is a true individual because of this union. However the child does obtain some genes from the father and the some from the mother. To complicate matters more some genes are dominant and some are recessive. The dominate ones express themselves with only one gene being present whereas the recessive genes require both of the genes to be present in order to be expressed; one from mother and one from father. Complicate this even further, there are some genes that are only partly dominant and some that are only partly recessive. The gender of the child was supposed to be the responsibility of the father's spermatozoa. However it has proved to be much more complicated than that. The mother's "egg" lives after its release, for the most for 24 hrs. Whereas spermatozoa do live at least 5 to7 days after they are released. It was believed that 'male' spermatozoa swam faster in the mother's birth canal; so that they arrived to the ovum sooner and hence the result was a male foetus. The female spermatozoa were believed to 'swim' slower and so would arrive a little later and then a female foetus would result from that conception. Male spermatozoa swim faster and so die sooner; female spermatozoa swim slower so they die later. So if conception occurred early and copulation occurred soon after ovulation and that conception happened; the result would result in a male foetus. Delaying copulation by several days would ensure that the male spermatozoa had died and female spermatozoa only survived hence a female foetus would result from that conception. So the timing copulation was supposed to give a much better chance of achieving the desired sex of the infant. At first systems were devised to time ovulation in order to select the gender of the child. Later the system developed as a system for birth control. (The Rhythm system of birth control), it was also referred to as the (Vatican Roulette). So for birth control, the time of copulation was to be avoided till at least 5 to 7 days after ovulation. This system was ok provided that the woman had regular periods. Many ways were developed to work out the time of ovulation; the best known one is the temperature method. I believe that a urine dip stick method has been developed to tell when copulation should not take place. There is such a thing as ovulation on demand as some women fund when their husbands came on leave during conflicts (wars) and they thought they were safe to have intercourse and the time was ok but they got pregnant anyway. Then there was a system using Vinegar (acidic) or bicarbonate of soda (alkaline) douches. The acidic douches were supposed to favour girl conceptions whereas alkaline douches were supposed to favour male foetuses. I think I do have it the right way around but in any case it did not work A Japanese company offered an expensive product that they could separate spermatozoa using electrophoresis thus using male spermatozoa or female spermatozoa to select the gender of the child you desired. All these systems don't work; but they did not guarantee it but they had your money anyway. The fact of the matter is that the whole issue is more complicated. We think now that it is probably the surface tension of the mother's egg that decides what sperm it will accept for fertilization. It is not the male partner that decides the gender of the child. It is even more complicated than that because there are families that have more boys than girls and vice versa. So it may be that the surface tension of the ovum is genetically determined. This is only a very brief and simplified 'lesson' on genetics. The study of genetics is very interesting and complicated.

I then go on to enquire about the mother's pregnancy with the presenting child; I enquire about the antenatal influences. Did she have ante natal care? What tests were done and what were the results of these tests; did she know the result of the tests? Did the mother take any medication during the identified patient pregnancy? Medications can include non-prescription medications. Often the mother does not think that they are medications because they are labelled heath food supplements; but in fact some do have interactions with medicine and are (legitimate) medications. For example St John wart is actually a mild SSRI (antidepressant). I ask about her alcohol intake during all her pregnancy; but especially during the first trimester of her pregnancy. I also enquire about her smoking during the pregnancy, (how many cigarettes did they smoke a day?) and what else do they admit to smoking. Did they suffer with high blood pressure or toxaemia? Did they have to be admitted to hospital because of these conditions, did they suffer with diabetes of pregnancy or just diabetes and was it monitored properly; and whether there were any other problems or complications during the pregnancy. A common problem during pregnancy is nausea, it is especially common during the first trimester; did they suffer from it and when did it stop? More importantly did they become dehydrated and did they require admission to hospital? . If it is not their first or only pregnancy a comparison with earlier other pregnancies may be useful.

I then go onto to ask about the actual delivery. Was it just normal? What was the length of the labour? Was the delivery complicated by any problem, were forceps used or was a vacuum extraction used? Was the delivery very quick? did the midwife call it a precipitated labour? This has to be asked directly because it is thought of as a good easy labour, but it can cause a problem to the infant. There are so many facts of the labour to ask about. Was there any dehydration occur during labour? Were there as enough nutrients (Sugar) during labour? Was there a drip running to provide essential nutrient and fluids? It is now customary to have a drip running during labour but it was not so years ago. Were there any complications? Such as eclampsia, did the labour had to be brought on (induced)? Was it an instrumental delivery and why was it necessary? Was the baby delivered by Caesarean Section? Was the Caesarean Section an emergency Caesarean or was it elective. What were the reasons that a Caesarean was done? As you can see there are many questions that need to be considered. Many children that have ADHD have a horrible birth history hence the original name of Minimal Brain Damage. I then proceed asking the mother about the child's history. I do start with the neonatal period. Was the child active right away; was the child normal at birth?

At the time of birth, the midwife 'measures' the child with what is called an Apgar score; It stands for American, Pediatric Gross Assessment Record, The nurse measures the .appearance-colour, pulse, grimace (reflex activity) the muscle tone. Do the parents remember the score? What was it? These bits of information do help to make a diagnosis, however do remember that very little can be done about these facts <u>now</u> but you and the family members can use these facts to make mothers feel guilt over the diagnosis. So be very alert not to do so!

The child's early development details are often available in the baby books; however many mothers forget to bring them in. In any case most mothers do recall many of the details! It never fails to amaze me how well mothers recall the individual child's details even when they have several children of different age to be concerned about.

I proceed further with the child's developmental history. When did they achieve their "milestones?" There are volumes written about children's milestones and the average age that children normally achieve these "mile stone". When did the child start holding their head up? When did they start smiling? Crawling? Walking? Talking? Speaking clearly? Placing words together? Talking in phrases and progressing to speak in sentences and so on. When were they toilet trained; both for bladder and bowels both day and night? Were these milestones on time or delayed? Did the child suffer with any trauma head or otherwise? Was the child ever unconscious and if so for how long, why had the child become unconscious? Had the child suffered meningitis? Did they go to preschool? Did they relate well and share their toys? At what age did they start school? How did the child progress at school? What was their behaviour like at school? There are so many questions. Was the child very oppositional? There is a variant of ADHD that is present in child hood and it is called Oppositional Defiant Behavior. A comparison to a sibling's development at a similar age may be very useful.

Then I proceed with their social development; how did they share their toy after 3, how they related to their peers, to the opposite sex, to adults and to authority. It is important to know how they communicated and related to various people that they came in contact with. What are their schools results like? How many schools did they attend? Did they have any problem and if so how was it dealt with? If they are older what progress was there in High school? How do they spend their spare time? What ambition do they have? What is the usual Dinner routine? How much time do they spend on the computer? How tidy is their room? What do they do in their room? Are they a clean "freak"? What social sites do they go to on their internet? Do the parents know what sites they go onto? What are their friends like, do the parent approve or disapprove of them and why? How many friends do they have? Are they invited to their friends' parties? Do they complete their tasks? Do they have problems sitting still? Do they have any problems with their concentration? Do they have any learning problems? What is their memory for school work like? Do they belong to any sporting club? Do they play an instrument? What music do they like? Do they stick at something? Do they take things apart and forget how they go together or just forget to put them back together? How happy they? Do they have any problem with their bowels or bladder? Have they strange eating habits, such as always wanting sugar? The older the "child is the more questions queries there are. With teenagers it is especially important to know if they are taking or smoking illicit drugs. It is interesting to read that many children start their alcohol or drug taking history when they are still in primary school. It does sound a bit like an inquisition however parents usually go straight to the details of their relevant concerns with their child and so many questions are already obvious that they don't have to be asked. However it is sometimes necessary, to ask specific questions, in order to make sure that all the correct details are obtained. It is important to be sure that the mother understand that the questions are being asked to help to make the diagnosis and they are not meant to be judgmental and thereby increase her guilt feelings and possibly make the child's self esteem worse. You need to be aware that the mother might already feel responsible in some way. I do use the time as an opportunity to reaffirm that they were not in a position to change certain factors now.

As I said earlier, a child diagnosed with ADD was believed to be due to some sort of brain damage. Occasionally there is a history of such a trauma. Nowadays it is well known to be due to a number of factors. Trauma, hereditary factors, birth injury including labour problems, mother's drinking or smoking (cigarettes or other substances), during pregnancy, and a variety of other problems are believed to be responsible. Nobody is really sure for certain, what is the root cause of these conditions.

Research has shown that in the majority of cases of Cerebral Palsy, it is because of some abnormality in the fetus that causes the birth defect. This fact is still ignored by the courts. The cause of all children born with Cerebral palsy is attributed to birth injury and often litigations do succeeds. The Victim often get large payouts-compensation for "birth injury", I suppose the courts want the child to be looked after; Centre link payments are insufficient for that purpose, so the courts make Medical Protection insurances societies pay. Certainly these unfortunate children and their family need help. But it does seem unfair that the medical profession is left to care for them. This has led to so many Medical Protection Societies going broke. It has been finally sorted out by our present prime minister. Many doctors find medical insurance premiums are prohibitive; many doctors and specialist don't practice high risks specialities such as delivering babies and neurosurgery in private practice any more. I have to continue to pay a "run out" insurance premium for several more years yet; this premium is on top of the basic cover premium. It is to cover the potential costs of any future suing. There are other far reaching consequences to the practice. Some "country" women find that they now have to travel from their home town for their deliveries; as their local doctor no longer deliver babies. Most doctors cannot justify the high premiums for a few deliveries. I know of several very good Obstetricians that only do Gynaecology in their private practice and have given up private obstetrics practice. The fees for private deliveries has increased to reflect those changes There is of no doubt that there are some cases of ADHD are due to brain damage, but they are in the small minority.

I will now go on to describe the examination of the child. The examination starts by observing the identified patient in the waiting room. They are observed as to how they relate to their family, (especially their mother), any other patients; both adults and children; that may be in the waiting room at the time of their appointment. (Hopefully I was not too late and the patient doesn't become very bored). The Child is observed how they interact with the receptionist and especially to the questions she asks of them. How they play, read and how they mix with other children in the waiting room. Remember that some of the other children that are in the waiting room are there because they too have various problems including some that may have ADHD or (Asperger's syndrome) themselves. The patient's reaction to those children has to be considered in the light of the other's child's condition. Were they shy? How they did play with other children? Were they anxious? How active were they? This may be how they are usually; it may be due to certain other factors; their behaviours and reactions have to be checked with the child's parents if they do react that way usually;. They may have been quite because they had preconceived expectations about coming to see a doctor and it may point to their anxiety. In my day, the doctor often was related to fear of needles. My parents would say things like 'if you don't behave you will have go to see the doctor'. Were they comfortable relating to other people? Did they child go to the parent and which on did they go to? Did the parents sit together? How directive was a parent? The observations of my receptionists, (which was usually my wife), and of myself are invaluable to make the diagnosis. A child, presented with an interesting and novel situation (toy often) may seem to concentrate well. It can be that they are so interested in the toy that they seemed to concentrate so well. There may also have been a chemical reason. A very interesting Canadian research did explain why many active children present as if they are quite, and butter would not melt in their mouths. They demonstrated, by with a blood test, that when the child is anxious; like when visiting a doctor, even that they do know the doctor well; they had a higher level of adrenalin in their circulation. Adrenalin is a stimulant hormone' like Ritalin is; hence the controlled behaviour. The parents become quite frustration when they tell the doctor how active their child is and their child is such an angel at the time of the consultation. They feel that you may not believe what they described about their child's activity. I often have to tell them of that important research that can explain why their child was appeared so well behaved and not active at their first examination; and not to worry as I will see their child's usual activity. I do often stir the child up to see their activity; I then observe how long it takes them to settle down. Children with features of ADHD take a long time to settle. The parents often 'thank me' for getting their child "so high". But they are happy (and relieved) that I can see how active their child can be! I may purposely leave the child to get bored by not providing them with any toy or any attention while I speak to the parents; I do this in order to see how they handle boredom. ADHD children handle boredom poorly. As I have mentioned already; there are far more distractions in the school classroom than there are in the consulting room; this factor needs to be considered. As an example of what is in most classrooms of today there are has many other children, so much going on in a class room, there are so many pictures, children's drawings, and all the other information pinned the class room walls. A subsequent interview may be necessary because of I may not see the child's distractibility in my waiting room as the child's teacher and parents) reported because of all the distractions in the classroom (and at home) as compared to my waiting room and the consultation room; they are so different that.

It is very important to establish rapport (if it is possible) with the child right away, so as to reduce any anxiety the child may have. If you fail to gain the child's confidence right away, it will prove a lot harder to obtain their trust later. The surgery waiting room and consultation room have to be child "friendly". It must have toys and children's books; including coloring in books and the materials to colour in with. It must contain material interesting to all ages for example adolescents and adults too. We keep the crayons and coloured pencils behind the reception desk and provide them to the children that request them.

The staff has to be used to, and be very comfortable with children of all ages. My wife was the practice manager and she is a great asset when it comes to making children comfortable. She has a skill, to talk to them and gain their confidence. We have 5 children, so she has had a lot experience in dealing with children. There is a wealth of invaluable observation both of the child and of the parents that must be made at the start of the consultation. The parents' ways are also to observed and noted. These are not for the purpose of being judgmental but to usefully arrive at the diagnosis and later to design management plan and advice. One or other parent may be ineffective, on the other end of the spectrum, one or other of the parents may be quite controlling, obsessive or even abusive or aggressive. The child's response may be submissive on the other hand they may be quite rebellious. In some cases the mother's may fuss over the child; in some cases of ADD or ADHD, the mother or (father) has hover over the child if they want anything done. The children get so distracted; that they don't complete anything- even getting dressed. One the other hand a parent may be referred to as a 'helicopter parent' it is the mother usually that unnecessarily fusses; they are always behind the child with directions; like be careful, don't climb the fence as you can fall down etc. etc.. Some mothers may tidy the toys in the waiting room before they come into the consultation room, or tell the child not to make a mess and to clean up. Mind you they may have to be so with very forgetful ADHD children. One has to be sure not to arrive to a wrong conclusion; one has to be sure if it is necessary for the child or it is the mother's personality? Repeated observations may be necessary; before a firm conclusion can be drawn. I have to be quite flexible and weigh things up as the situation presents. I prefer to initially see adolescents on their own; they nearly always feel more at ease on their own. With young children, I invite the child and the family to come into my consulting room. I consider it very, very important to try and put patient and the parents at ease, straight away. Coming to a consultation can be is very harrowing an experience for both child and parents of itself. Often they may already have had several consultations with various other practitioner's; which may not have been satisfactory experiences. Some children may have been 'over doctors' by over concerned parents.. Some children have had previous bad experiences like painful injections or some other treatment, so they are frightened and upset from the start. Often their upset can be traced back to some bad experience that they had with a doctor in the past-or that they may suffer with anxiety problems.

I have said previously, the referrals do come from various agencies. Occasionally, they parents have forgotten to bring the referral letter to the appointment, usually the parents themselves are able to provide me with the reason for the referral and I try do remind them to bring it when they come for the next the appointment. In case there may have been some important facts in the letter that the parents forgot to tell me; either on purpose or they genuinely forgot. Some referrals provide very little information, they are worded something like- this "please assess this child!" I must admit I have been very slack in returning feedback letters to the referring agencies, although I do sometimes talk to them on the telephone. It is very important not to be judgmental or to be influenced by the agency that the referral comes from. I often contact the original referral agency if I do not see some patients again; that is all I can do as a private medical practitioner I don't have any more power than that.

Sometimes the referral comes from other agencies including a Psychiatrist often because a parent or parents are themselves going through some therapy. In Australia the availability of psychiatric treatment is at limited (at times). Under ideal circumstances, separate family members undergoing therapy should see separate therapists. However, at times, I found myself having to wear "several hats" as it were. One is for the first patient and for individual therapy, one for a second patient or another family member and a third for family therapy. I such cases it is very important to maintain confidentiality; (when seeing several people as it is important for their trust). At times it can be very difficult to maintain the privacy but it is of the utmost importance. I do sometimes get tested out; I would get accused of having said something I had not. You can imagine the dilemma, during those times it is very tempting to deny that I did in fact not say the thing I was accused of saying, I tactfully say that they know me well, so " would I betray your trust? " In most cases it does end up working ok. I'd often encourage patients to discuss their concerns with the other patients with similar problems. I will describe how well it does work with the parent (mothers) of the young children suspected of having ADHD. The comfort that they do get from talking to other parents that are confronted with the same or similar problems is heartening.

Children that have any problems, like ADD or ADHD often get poor school results. They often know that they are capable of better results, some are quite clever, but for their distractibility and their poor attention problems and organization ability and their probable unrecognized learning problems; results in that they don't achieve to their potential. I again emphasize; they often end up with a poor self esteem and they often end up having developed an associated behaviour problem. The circle usually begins by poor behaviour then rejection by our society; and then more behaviour problems and more poor self worth. Occasionally, the parents have a different opinion to the referral letter so it important to hear why they hold that opinion; even though the temptation is to wonder, if is it only because of their bias; that their opinions are often so different from the original (often teacher's letter-the concerns that were expressed in the referral letter. In most cases, the child's parents do know the child best however it may be because as I said it may be because they don't see their child at school. Most parents do seek help to get the best for their child.

I make sure that the child is allowed to have sweets as soon as the child enters my consulting room. That is because some children have been put on a diet and they are not allowed certain colouring or sweets, on the mistaken advice that this would help their child with ADHD. I will discuss the reason for my opinion later. If they are allowed sweets, I do offer them a one. It is wonderful to see how well lollies work to get them to relax and to gain their confidence. Thank God for lollies; they look forward to the sweets on subsequent appointments. Dentists do recommend that we brush our teeth after eating sweets, so I do encourage that they brush their teeth after eating lollies. If sweets are not enough a joke, (at their level), is often needed as well as the lollies to help them to relax. It is very important with any patient but especially so with anxious children that the patient is totally comfortable throughout the whole of the history taking and especially examination. The parents understand and appreciate it when they see their child relax. It is just as important that the parent feel at ease as their anxiety can be felt by the patient. I proceed then to enquire further about the child's history; was there a history of any taste or smell aberrations; such as the child loving things like sour foods or having a great liking of sweet things. The parents may recall that the child wanted to smell everything; this is a common feature of children with Asperger's syndrome. I'd also enquire about any history that they may choose inappropriate clothing for the weather. E.g.: the wearing of jumpers in summer. I'd then start with the formal examination; during the examination, especially of their private areas, one parent should/ must be present always; this protects the practitioner from accusations as well as relaxing the nervous child I start by measuring the child's weight and height and weight; many children are very interested in their measurements, especially the progressive measurements. I do encourage the children to be familiar with my examination instruments. I was nervous about them touching my instruments but in some almost 40 years of practice I have only had one instrument damaged in that time. I'd progress to examine their body. I would usually start with the head. I would feel the bony skull for any lumps or bumps; I would also measure the skull if it seemed to be too big or too small-micro or macro changes. I would go down the head by examining the lips, mouth, palate, (soft and hard), tongue, and the pharynx. The movement of the tongue and lips are checked I very rarely do find a case of a tongue tie or of soft cleft palate that has been missed, however it must be looked for. This examination is particularly important if speech and language problems are present. The back of the throat is usually pink however in cases such as vasomotor pharyngitis, which is associated nasal changes similar to allergic rhinitis when it is pale pink, glistening and often rough, like an orange skin. The nasal areas are examined for any signs of pallor and mucous; these may point to vasomotor rhinitis which may be part of vasomotor nasopharyngeal irritation or of nasal allergy. Children with ADD and Aspergius syndrome often complain of nasal obstruction and allergy; this is only party responsive to antihistamines. Cases of vasomotor pharyngitis are common as they are a vasomotor phenomenon. I will speak later of one treatment for ADHD which is a blood pressure medication which may sometimes be useful for ADHD and for this condition. The nasal examination is easy to do, and it is very informative. I'd use the light of an auto scope. The children often refer to this instrument as a "nasal looker inner". The nasal mucosa is usually pinkish red. But in children with the condition of vasomotor rhinitis the nasal mucosa is not the usual red but it is pink, glistening and full of mucous. The bony features in the nose create a vortex when air is breathed through the nose thereby precipitating material in the air and at the same time heating the incoming air. They are called the bony turbinate's. The mucous membrane becomes swollen and the mucous exudates collect.

I believe that it is why some nutritionist or dieticians believe that it is because of this feature that mimics allergies that food sensitivities are often believed to be responsible for the condition of ADD or ADHD. They write books and design diets that restrict certain foods that contain the naturally occurring or artificially obtained salicylates; they are supposed to cause several of the symptoms of ADHD. There is a lot of evidence that does not support these diet is responsible for many of the symptoms and signs of ADHD. In a few cases only, and certainly only a few cases of the allergic condition is undeniably present. It may be associated to ADHD but it can be present anyway. If the allergy does exist then the elimination of the allergen is necessary; however the fundamental condition of ADHD is not controlled by this diet. I would like to quote a research that was undertaken in the United States of America. A city with the population of a hundred thousand people was chosen for the research study. The whole diet of the city was controlled so that a main frame computer that "knew" what food would be consumed by the children studied, even the food that that children studied could access was known by the computer. Children often do swap lunches etc. so it was important to know what food the children had access to. The observers reported on individual's children's behaviours and activity. Remember that the observers did not know what child was on the diet and what child was not on the diet. In this way bias was eliminated. At the conclusion of the study the researches could not find any correlation to any food sensitivity. Even Australia's own NHMRC (Nation Health and Medical Research Council) published a paper some years ago stating that they could not find any evidence supporting the claim that the diet affected the behaviour of ADHD. I will elaborate further on diets later..

When the child has a lot of nasal obstruction the possibility of sleep apnea has to be thought of; I must admit I rarely look into it, because I'd rarely think of it. Often the parents have already had the child's hearing tested; as it is one of the first things that most parent do when they are confronted that their child has learning problems. I do however test their hearing myself. I start to examine the ears by looking at the ear drum using an autoscore. I'd often see the elderly with wax in their ear canal that affected their hearing but I would very rarely see kids with such a problem. If the hearing is affected because the wax totally obstructs the external canal than an ear syringe easily corrects this problem. Sometimes it does take a few days inserting oily drops to soften the wax before the ear is syringed is effective.

The ear drum is usually almost transparent and pale pink; and you can see the shadows of the bones in the middle ear; however it can be very dull, if the middle ear is full of mucous or it can be red if it is infected. . The diameter of the Estuation tube is too little in early child hood, as it will not allow for the drainage of thick mucus; which is the left over generally results from an ear infection. Ear infections are common enough with young children. Although it the ear infections do eventually heal up; the thick muocus that cannot drain does affect the conductive hearing of the child which in turn affects their speech and language development and then causes learning problems. Children then need the help of a pediatric ENT surgeon to insert Grommets so that the thick mucous is drained and their hearing development etc. is normal. I'd proceed then to check the child's normal hearing; I'd ask that everyone in the room to be very quiet, then I'd whisper very quietly in each of the patient ears in turn, first in one ear and then the in the other. I'd increase the loudness of whisper until they hear me clearly. I'd then ask the people in the room to talk while I'd repeat the hearing test to assess how their hearing is with back ground noise. This problem is more often observed with the elderly but very occasionally it presents with the ADHD child. If the child in question does have such a problem it must present a problem for the child in a noisy class room. If I was in doubt about the child's hearing I'd do use a tuning fork. The tuning fork is used to test bony hearing and conduction hearing. The tuning fork is started to vibrate and then I ask the child to listen to it. When they stop hearing it I place it on the bony feature, just behind their ear; if they can hear it then; it does mean they do have a conduction hearing loss; alternative; I start the tuning fork vibrating; I place the tuning fork on the bony area behind their ear first and then ask them to tell when they stop hearing the tuning fork making a sound. I then listen to it if I can still hear it then the child has a hearing loss. Very occasionally I do see an older child that has been missed; they have fluid in the middle ear. Normal hearing is so important that if any doubt exist about the child's hearing, an ENT referral is mandatory. I'd move down the child's neck next, and I start to look at the thyroid gland. I look for any lumps or enlargement. In the past a cause of severe mental retardation was the result of an underactive thyroid. The retardation can be prevented if the problem is discovered early. Nowadays the thyroid function is tested for soon after birth; most are tested even before the child leaves hospital (by a heal prick). It is very important to diagnose this condition as early as possible; because the changes are irreversible and the child is left with retardation. I do worry that as and if the 'home births' become more prominent; that if this test is missed we could go back to days; when we had more cases of mental retardation because this test was neglected and not conducted.. Incidentally, the thyroid gland adjusts or metabolism to cope with the weather condition; however it does take some three month to do so. I rarely find any problem with the thyroid as I do with the normal examination. I'd then examine the neck for enlarged lymphatic glands. I do start with the tonsillar glands. These are at the angle of the jaw, they are often present and they are slightly enlarged in most children. These glands don't mean that much is wrong as they are they are the factories, as it were, that make the antibodies to fight infections. If they are grossly enlarged they may point out to a chronic infection or something more sinister. In the case that they are soft, then the infection is current. They do appear hard if the infection has gone. The other sites that these lymphatic glands are found include the axilla (arm pits) and the groins. So while looking at the glands I look at these other sites. Very occasionally these enlarged glands may point to other very sinister problems such as leukaemia. There are other sites that may contain these glands; for an example the post cervical glands. They too have to be examined. Incidentally the old fashion of tonsillectomy (removal of the tonsils has been discontinued). The tonsils are the first line of defence for the lung so the unnecessary removal of them can result in the child getting asthma; naturally, badly infected pussy ones do have to be removed.

The breathing is examined using a percussion of the chest; percussion is performed by placing ones fingers on the chest wall and using the fingers of the other hand to knock on them; then listening to the sound that that makes. The chest is an air filled chamber so the sound it makes is that of a hollow area, if the sound is dull; like that of a solid area; it is abnormal. Listening to the lungs by using a stethoscope can support the abnormal findings; I would then order a chest x ray to support my diagnosis. It is extremely rare that such an abnormal finding is found. The shape of the chest is noted. I have seen both pigeon and cavous deformities of the chest. Even though they do look dreadful these deformities very rarely cause a problem

I'd listen to the heart. The heart sounds are due to the flow of blood across the heart valves. I especially listen to those sounds. I have come across abnormalities that are picked up through the heart sounds. After first discussing with parents and making sure that the understand the exactly the reasons for the consultation and not dramatically presenting the problem and increasing their anxiety unnecessarily I'd obtain a paediatric consultation, either with a paediatrician of their choice or if they do not have one, I arrange either a private consultation or a consultation through a public hospital outpatient.

I'd examine the abdomen next. I enquire about reflux symptoms; mind you children that don't know any better often accept symptoms as normal and have not complained to the parents; when I do ask about the symptom it is only then that most the children realize it is not normal to suffer these symptoms.. I'd feel for any enlargement of the liver and spleen. I do feel for any faecal masses in the abdomen. One cannot usually feel any faecal material in the lower bowel. These faecal lumps point to chronic constipation.

Children with ADD or Asperger's syndrome often suffer with chronic constipation.

I look at the skeletal system next; I start by looking at the back. I look for any curvature or twisting of the spine. I'd look at the joints for any abnormalities. Occasionally there is a difference of leg lengths. Any abnormalities in those examinations require the appropriate referral. Again I'd ensure that the parents and the child understand fully the reasons for the referral and ensure that unnecessary anxiety results because of the referral. I look at the skin and I take note of any abnormal moles or lesions.

I'd then do a neurological screen. During this part of the examination I look at the child's gait, tone, their muscular power and their reflexes. These reflexes include the biceps, triceps, knee, ankle jerks, the planter's and the reflex called the Babinski reflex. This reflex is tested by stimulating the shin of each leg in turn and watching the response of the toes of the same leg, both the planters and the Babinski reflexes do rarely point to a problem in children brain; but they more commonly wrong in the elderly. The plantar reflexes are done by rubbing the sole of the feet and watching what the toes do. The toes usually go down going as you rub the sole of the foot; another way to get a similar response is to rub the shin of the lower leg down wards; if there is something very wrong with neurological function the toes may be up going. I'd do a test that is known as the Romberg's test. The child is asked to stand up and get their balance once they are balanced they are asked to close their eyes and their balance is again observed. I then do a test to check their fine coordination; it is called the finger nose test it is done by asking the patient to stand about a foot away from me then to touch my nose with their index finger of their dominant hand; then they quickly touch their own nose with the same index finger and back to my nose quickly and so on; I repeat the test with their eyes opened and their eyes closed. I then ask them to change hands, still with their eyes closed. Usually the patient would open their eyes so I have to start all over again. I very rarely find any problem with children; but I do the full examination anyway. Very occasionally I do get a surprise and find a problem.

If a neurological problem is suspected a neurological referral is needed. A neurologist, often a paediatric neurologist or one that is experienced with children, is chosen for this referral. Often an examination and an E.E.G. (electro encephalogram) are ordered by the neurologist; E.E.G. is traced with some simulation for example their eyes open and then closed. Many children loved this test as they had to have a good blood sugar level at the time of the test so I would tell their mother to give them a sweet drink or a chocolate bar just before they had their test. Children with ADHD often have slight differences (non specific changes) on their EEG traces. That is probably why it was earlier believed that children ADHD had "minimal brain damage". In fact ADHD was initially called "minimal brain damage" and later it was called "minimal brain dysfunction" before it was appropriately called ADHD. Although E.E.Gs, were often done previously for children with ADHD they often only showed non-specific abnormalities so nowadays they are not ordered much. An EEG will show up any abnormality of the brains electrical activity so they are very useful for 'electrical abnormities' as are seen in epilepsy. Children with explosive tempers are suspected of suffering with Temporal lobe epilepsy so EEG's are the test of choice; however, occasionally a sleep EEG is requested. As a normal EEG may not show the abnormality Again I want to emphasis that although I do the normal physical examination; I very rare do find any problem besides vasomotor rhinitis and signs of constipation. After this part of the formal examination is complete I'd often ask the child if they would like to take a break and go into the shop and get a drink or a small treat before we go on with the rest of the assessment. I am in fact continuing with the examination. I always find that this suggestion is very welcomed by the children. Some parents offer to pay for the treat but I do explain that is my treat as the child has been so good and co-operated so well. I'd then add a slight condition to get their treat. The condition was to accept a 'piggyback' from me. The children do hesitate at first; until they heard what the condition is; most children then eagerly accept the 'piggyback'. Many children look forward to their follow up appointment as they ask me if they can have another piggy back. Some, young children, are very anxious and balk at the thought of a "piggy back". So if a child does not want to, I don't insist. However, I do try to encourage them, luckily, one way or another, 'touch wood', it always worked out.

Once, in over 30 years of practice I was accused of being some sort of a paedophile! The parent did not say anything at the time of the assessment. The parents wrote to The Director General of Health complaining that I was a paedophile because I wanted to give their child a piggy back. The Director of Health wrote to me for an explanation. I understand he had to take some action to a formal complaint no matter how frivolous it is. Careful explanation as to why I did these things resolved the departments concerns. The shoulder ride offers me a good chance for many more observations. As I take the child to the local shop I first observed the child's balance; as I'd playfully twist from side to side I pretend to fall. I can see how they adjust their balance to cope with my changing their balance, and how quickly they do change their centre of gravity to cope with my changing their balance; I can see if they are fearful of falling. As I go down some stairs I'd observed if they had a fear of heights; I get a feel of how anxious they are. The local shop used to be just next door; but it closed down so now I have to take the child across the road to another shop. At first I thought it was a concern but as it has turned out it allows for more observation; the way they walk or just run; I'd see the evidence of their activity (or their hyperactivity); the way they obeyed the traffic lights; the way they listened to my instructions while crossing the road; when they had to accept to hold my hand crossing the road. It can be very informative to see the child outside of the consultation room. I'd listen to them and observe how they may be different when, and away from their parents. Perhaps that is evidence of an anxious and over controlling parent. At the shop they, are allowed to choose a small treat. This also allows for very valuable and useful observation. Do they accept limits? How pleasant were they to the shop keeper? What is their money sense like? How do they work out what change should they get? Is their maths ability appropriate to their age? Does is the child overcome by so many choices? Were they "distracted" by so many choices? Were they decisive? Were they undecided when they were presented with so many choices? Some children try to bargain with me about the limit that I offered them. It is interesting to watch the Asperger's child that was generally anxious becoming outgoing and bargaining with a shop keeper to get quite a discount on an item they wanted; but it did cost more than the limit I had set them; they first tried bargain with me about the limit I had given them; when that failed they turned to the shopkeeper to try and get the item that they wanted for less. Some children were particularly persistent in contrast to what I had seen of their behaviour previously. What in fact their usual behaviour? There is a wealth of observation that has to be made before the correct diagnosis is arrived at. I have only mentioned some of the observations that I do make. Sometimes I wonder how it is that some practitioners can make an informed diagnosis without these observations in the many different situations; I can't understand how one can see what a child's is really like if the child gets to sit with a new, novel and interesting toy; in a waiting room or a consultation room and judge that their concentration is good. They may seem be so interested; that they seem to be able to concentrate well. Parents tell me that there are times that they cannot pull their child away from what they may be really interested with; they may find it so difficult to believe when other people tell them that their child can't concentrate because they cannot get their child off the play station that their child is fascinated with. Their relationship ability is often judged one interview also. I do realize that experience is invaluable; however ADHD or Asperger's syndrome children are so different in different times at in different situations that some children require more than one examination to make a final diagnosis. In certain case, a once only examination is not enough to make a definitive diagnosis and to prescribe the correct treatment; although it so happens that in the majority of cases a diagnosis and prescription of the correct treatment is arrived at after one long consultation. One should not assume that the parents and child (adolescent) should just accept the diagnosis. Perhaps that it was the way it was years ago, that they just accepted the doctor's diagnosis. Let me remind you of the experience that I had when I did a locum in Geelong. The patient's notes indicated that their prescription were for red pills, blue pills etc. I waited anxiously for the principal's arrival; he was not even out of the car when I raced over to him and asked what these coloured pills were that I had prescribed. He told me not to worry they were only vitamins. Then he added that if patients believed enough that they would help they did help, (they did). Now day's parents do required more explanation for their child and their own treatments, lest they will consult professor Google or to god know who. This will ensure that they will be more confused by the information and opinions that the various sites give them. Some opinions will be very biased.

Let's return now to the observations that I do make. On our way back from the shop it is very useful opportunity to obtain more information, such as their relationship with siblings and parents is? Their perception of how strict the school is; how strict their parents are? what are their interests; what they eventually hope to be; there are their views of the attitudes of their parents, to them and their other siblings, their view of school and school admiration; if they belong to sporting or and other clubs; their opinion of their sports leaders. I watch see what their awareness of traffic, how they obey traffic rules and what their road sense is like, etc. I do not "pump" them for information, but I listen to their spontaneous conversations and only if they don't spontaneous tell me things I will gently question them.

I think it is worth recounting the following incident as it demonstrates two important aspects. One is the anxiety that Asperger's syndrome children have and the other is the vigilance that people should have to prevent abduction of children by predators. On one occasion, during a follow up consultation, I was taking a boy diagnosed with Asperger's syndrome who was very anxious to the shop; His condition was complicated by a very controlling father. As we were crossing the main road to go to the shop, he saw a police car, he to froze in the middle of the road. I had no choice, as the traffic lights were about to change to red; I held his hand firmly and I pulled him across the road. A passing motorist was vigilant enough, and thought that I was forcing this boy; he stopped his car and accosted me till he called the police. I have practiced in Kallangur for many years so the locals knew me well, however he would not be reassured by them, until the police arrived and interview me. On one hand, I was pleased that he was concerned enough to follow his instinct, however, one the other hand, I do wish he would have listened to the locals. The reaction that the boy had was really bad. He was sweating, almost shaking and very upset. He really did think that he was in trouble; that the police were there for him. It is amazing how children can misinterpret incidences, that is especially so with Asperger's syndrome but also with very many children. In any case, all it all ended well. When we return from the shop I'd get the child to eat their treat or play with the toy that they chose their treat that they purchased from the shop. I then ask the parents more questions. I have described that sometimes I allow the child to get bored to observe their reaction. I may ask other professional for more help. A psychologist can to help to clarify formally and confirm my opinions accurately; they can further assess their ability and perception including any learning problems and features of their personality like, depression, anxiety and their emotional state. Children suffer from all grades of depression. I know of a child that I suspect hung himself. It was put down to accidentally having been hung on a clothes line. We now do know that a major cause of child suicide is bulling. Speech therapists (or their new name is speech pathologist) are involved to formally assess a speech and language disorder; an occupational therapists is often involved in the child's treatment; for an example bowel problems.

Sensory Motor Examination

I will describe this screening examination. This Sensory Motor Examination is often much more fruitful than the traditional physical examination. This examination looks for the so called "soft signs". These sign are, in isolation of not of much significance, however in association with each other signs do mean a lot. They point to a diagnosis of ADHD. I have already described a small part of that examination (for instance balance) when I talked about the observations that I'd made during the "piggy back".. As I describe the sensory motor examination; I will go further and try to explain what many of these "soft signs" can mean. Our bodies have seven sensory inputs. They are- (1).Gustatory- tastes (2).Olfactory- smell. (3). Tactile- feelings with the four divisions, soft touch, pain, vibration and temperature, not absolute temperature but changes of temperature, vision (4).Visual-sight (5).Auditory- (6).Vestibular- (7).Propioception-body sense. All the information from these senses integrates. The information inputs from these inputs are then stores using the memory modality; this enables us to be able to store the input information.

I will present the "model "that use and that I have developed to explain and understand this process better.

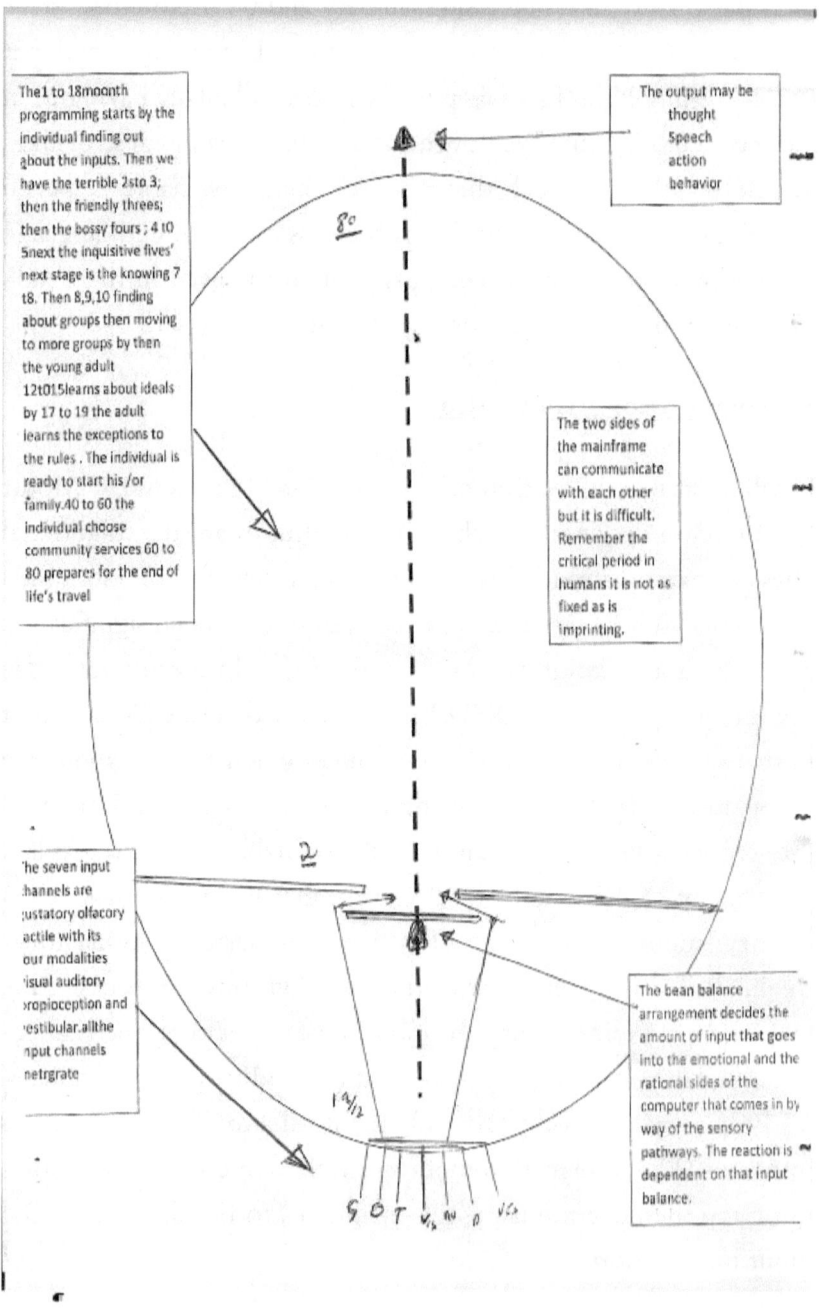

The1 to 18moonth programming starts by the individual finding out about the inputs. Then we have the terrible 2sto 3; then the friendly threes; then the bossy fours ; 4 t0 5next the inquisitive fives' next stage is the knowing 7 t8. Then 8,9,10 finding about groups then moving to more groups by then the young adult 12t015learns about ideals by 17 to 19 the adult learns the exceptions to the rules . The individual is ready to start his /or family.40 to 60 the individual choose community services 60 to 80 prepares for the end of life's travel

The output may be thought Speech action behavior

The two sides of the mainframe can communicate with each other but it is difficult. Remember the critical period in humans it is not as fixed as is imprinting.

'he seven input channels are :ustatory olfacory actile with its our modalities 'isual auditory :ropioception and 'estibular.allthe nput channels netrgrate

The bean balance arrangement decides the amount of input that goes into the emotional and the rational sides of the computer that comes in by way of the sensory pathways. The reaction is dependent on that input balance.

All the sensory organ pathways have to be examined carefully as so are the memory aspects.

The gustatory tastes sense is of interest because several of the parents' of ADHD children do reported that their children have weird tastes; for instance they like things that are sickly sweet or very sour.

The Olfactory sensation (smell) doesn't seem to occupy as big an area in the human brain as it does occupy in certain animals; like in canines (dog). Many Asperger's children like to smell things. The sense of taste and smell are of interest and are enquired about, but I don't test for them specifically.

The Tactile system. We have already observed during the normal physical examination that the child was excessively ticklish or loathed being touched and we heard; during the history taking that some children chose inappropriate clothing for the prevailing weather

The Visual pathway consists of many aspects. These include visual acuity, which we think about when we talk of eye sight. Many children have had their eyes tested already; the parents of children that have reading problems often take their child to an optometrist to have an eye test. However, the child with ADHD rarely has visual acuity defects at least no more than the general population does. I do test the child's visual acuity if it has not been already been tested.

Diverting a little; it was the ophthalmologists that first described learning problems because of what is now known to be because of visual perceptual problems. At one stage a dramatic report with a "fun fare" that coloured glasses corrected many of the reading problems. Alas, the coloured glasses were another expensive disappointment for the parents that hoped they had found the answer to their child's learning problem. I'd do test the child's color vision using the Ishihara charts for color vision. I'd occasionally find a defect but it very rarely but if ever, it causes a reading problem. I will now describe the many problems that arise because of visual perception problems; reading is such a complex skill; most of us take the reading skill for granted. I generally start by testing their reading skill. I do use reading tests; these reading tests are used to measure the child's reading level; I use the St Lucia reading test older children (it was developed in Queensland), I find the Hull B test is useful for the younger child. Both these tests provide 'Age' levels so that their reading level can be compared to their age. Both these tests are readily available on the internet. If I do suspect reading perceptual problems I proceed to look further into the perceptual problems. Maybe because I still have problems in that area!

I'd use charts like the Frostig diagrams to assess the perceptual problems that the child may have. These charts are available on the internet but I have 'borrowed' them that from a psychologist. There exists a Marianne Institute in the USA. That institute developed the visual perception tests that are so useful. I will now describe some of these test charts. One chart shows a tree with a bird on the left branch of the tree and the other 4 or 5 picture the bird is on a right branch. The child is asked to point to the only one that the bird is on the left branch but of course they are not given the clue; they are just asked to find the only figure that is different. In another chart, the picture is of 5 elephants with their trunks in the direction of the left side but only one pointing his trunk to the right direction. Again the child is asked to point to the only one that is different!

The charts are be further complicated by the different the size of the bird; with or different sized of the elephant trunk. I have not had to use these more complicated ones as I usually observe the problems that some children have with the initial charts! This is a test to assess the child's sense of direction. I will later describe how the sense direction is so important for a child to be able to read words. In another picture there certain parts of the picture missing for instance a three legged table. This test relies on the child's memory of what the object should look like. The child is presented with a picture of three objects and asked to find the similarities of two of them; for an example the pictures are of a basket a tree and an umbrella. Is the tree has fiber as is the basket made of? There are several answers to the question; the child's task is to come up with an answer that makes sense! This tests the child's ability to associate things. Another picture is used to tests the child's sense of humour. The picture is of person (usually a girl child) fishing; however they pull up an old tyre; Can they focus their ability on what is asked of them? Can they focus on the funny part of the picture? I'd ask the older children to copy a complex diagram which involves several lines, shapes and angles. All the aspects of visual perception have to be tested; some of these include shape constancy, visual direction of symbols, including rotations, or mirror reversals, closing of visual symbols, sequencing, and off course the visual memory aspects cannot be ignored. The problems that occur in the visual pathways have so many features to consider.

Let's start by looking at shape constancy. A good example of this is demonstrated by considering that the eyes can interpret that a small b is actually the same symbol as a B. Yet the brain should be able to recognize that they are indeed the same Next we have to understand the complexity that our ability to understand the coding that our alphabet and in turn our reading depend upon. Let's start mirror imaging our symbols; does not a 5 look like the mirror image of a five. A 2 like the mirror image of a two. Take the example of a q then look at p are they not the mirror images of the same symbol? If you replace a p by a q is it the same word then? Let's complicate this further by rotating the symbol by 90 degrees. Do a c and a u look alike (apart from the curves)? Are they really the same? Now let us rotate the symbol some180 degrees; invert the symbols w, m. are they the same? What if the child sees them as the same symbol? Now let's understand a further possible difficulty, a child may have; difficulty with closures of symbols. Take the example of this problem that a child can have is demonstrated by the following; take the letter a, how much different is it with the letter n? If the bottom of the letter is left open; if the symbol is not closed, is in fact the same? If the length of upstroke is not easily perceived, is it an n like a or h?

Now let's complicate this further by combining letters that have been perceived wrongly. Let's say that the letters were incorrectly perceived, does what the child reads make sense? Will complications of perception not lead to further problems? Now complicate their problem using the whole word. If they do easily reverse symbols then was can be "seen" as saw? Does dog not look different to god? Are bed and deb, nat and hat the same? Can you see what can go wrong, and what difficulty that a child has with visual perceptual problems, when it come to reading? Make it even more complex; to visual perception problems add auditory perceptual problems and them add memory problems- is it any wonder it is too much so the child just want to avoid such a reading difficulty? What a mess can result from such a confusing problem; they then get further behind by avoiding reading and they end up being further behind and so on (probably too far behind to catch up)! The visual images of the words are associated to the memory of the auditory pathways (the hearing pathway) so that they mean something; the stored memory related to what we are reading; to the sound of either an object or an action.

Hearing was already tested as I have described. As I whisper quietly in the child's ear, first in one ear then the other. They may confuse the words; it is unusually a hearing acuity problem; it is usually an auditory perception problem. Auditory perception enables us to recognize that the different sounds at various volumes that mean the same. The gaps between sounds have to be recognized if speech is to mean anything or if we do not all we hear is a continued jumble of sounds. If you listen a conversation between two people that are talking in a language that you don't know, you will see what I mean! The different accents can be another complication; they can be very difficult to understand. Evelyn is originally from Scotland. We were recently having lunch in a Scottish pub; even though when we started talking with very friendly local we could not understand anything he said to us until he changed to talking to us in kings English. This further needs all the memory tracts so that one remembers what those sounds mean. I will describe how I test some of the four the memory aspects. I do test the short term memory of a child by getting them to stand several feet away from me and then I callout out several numbers, colors or objects to them. I ask them to just wait till I have finished calling the numbers or objects or fruits or whatever interests the child; they just have to call them back to me (preferably) in the same order. If they don't get it the first time I'd repeat the test by using different numbers etc. The length of the list of numbers etc. depends on the age of the child. For an example the average 7 year old child will recall at least a series of 5 numbers. Usually they will also reply in the same order as they were called out to them. Many times, if I have to repeat the test by using a different set of numbers or object; I often get numbers or objects from the first list called out back to me- this usually points that the child has perseveration problems. I complicate this test further by asking them not only to recall the numbers but to call them out to reversing the numbers. E.g. 84531 they should call back 13548. I purposely get the order mixed up when I repeat the numbers to observe if they pick me up, most children seem to love picking me up when I make a mistake. The ones with memory problems are not the ones that pick me up as they are really unaware that I was incorrect. Many children with learning problems actually have <u>short term memory</u> problems as well. I'd often use a different test with older children to test their short term memory. I'd read them a list of several words (16) twice; then ask the child to recall as many of the words I'd had just read to them. I would often complicate this test further by reading a new list of words twice again and then ask them to recall as many of the words from the new list as they can recall but not giving me some words from the previous list. When they do remember words that were from the first list it indicates another problem of memory called perseveration problems.

We just all just take the reading skill for granted. You can gleam how minor problems in our <u>coding</u> skills can result in major difficulties in reading. The child with visual perception problems does have learning problems. Visual perception is such a delicate and complicated skill that it's a wonder that it does not go wrong more often; it is another wonder how the brain corrects part of the problem as time goes on. Complicate their problems further by adding problems in Auditory perception and memory problems and you can realize why the avoid reading- does the jumble of symbols and sound that don't mean anything really should mean something?

The Vestibular reception organ is located in the middle ear next to the hearing organ. There is one on either side. Each one consists of three semicircular canals placed in different planes. One is horizontal, one is vertical and the third is oblique. The canals are filled with inertia less fluid so that moment of the body especially the head moves in any direction the movement is registered; but as soon we stops so does the stimulation. Because the fluid is inertia less; any movement of the fluid stop moving as soon as the head stops moving. The movement of the fluid stimulates hair like receptor in the semicircular canals from both sides (organs); they in turn are associated to visual impulses so we know what is happening to our body's position at that time. This is a very simple explanation however the brain connection to the various centers is very complicated. Vision is involved as well as balance ; there are several nuclei involves as is the Cerebella nuclei The fluid in the canals can thicken with most infections; it then is no longer inertia less; it does returns to the inertia less condition but with some if it does not; as seen in vestibullitis; it can also be centrally activated. There is a genetic condition called Mernier's Disease in that the brain causes dizziness. It presents as we get older. Dizziness happened to me after I had Dengue fever in New Guinea. I told you about when my then five year old daughter jumped on my bed. The hearing organ also deteriorates as we get older as well. We then also suffer ringing in the ears called tinnitus. Can you recall the merry go rounds in our youth? They were common in our play grounds then. We would spin on them and be all dizzy when we hopped off! This is the reaction of stimulating by the vestibular organ.

In children this organ is very important as it is involved in providing our perception of the sense of direction. Remember that the direction of the symbols of letter and of words? How important they are? I test this organ by sitting the child on my office rotating chair. I would cover their eyes so that vision cannot compensate for this sense. I have clinically and empirically found that 5 spins are optimal to observe most children's reaction to spinning. I'd spin them on the chair reasonably fast, at first to one side and then the other to the side; I watch their eyes after I stop spinning them in either direction. I will describe the reactions later. The child demonstrates all manner of differences reactions to this testing. They can show extreme sensitivity and they get nausea with even just a gentle spin. I have to be very careful with such children (or they would end up vomiting) not to keep spinning them on the chair; when I do know from the history that the child hates spinning. Fortunately these children represent the minority.

With some children that don't show any response to spinning, I would spin them again. I'd spin them seven times and just as fast. Just as I stop them spinning I take their blind fold off and observe the reaction of their eyes. Just as I said; children can demonstrate different responses from spin in different directions. Their eyes move to the lateral side and back to the middle of their eyes as if trying to make sense of the spin. The 'nystagmus' can die off quickly, not happen at all, or go on for a long time. It can occur at different speeds and different in the different direction of spin. I'd often use this test, on its own, to assess the progress of treatment. I'd show parents the result of this test many a time; so that they could see for themselves what I was talking about. Any test should be fun for the child so at the end of this test I usually pretend to make the chair fall backwards. Most children love that so much so that they ask me to do it again at subsequent appointments. It was very encouraging that they felt so comfortable in the surgery that they can confidently ask me to do the things that they like.

The Propioception sense.

This skill is tested by first covering the child's eyes and then I ask them to give me one hand. I'd then touch one finger and then ask them to identify the finger I had touched. They then show me the finger I touched, or name the finger I touched or just move that finger. I then touch a different finger and so on. If I suspected a problem in this area I'd touch several places on the same finger. Often children find the 4th finger is more difficult to identify. Children like it when I touch their middle finger and they can then are able to give me the rude "finger" without being told off. I then repeat the test with the other hand. I showed the father from the group Father's caring for kids and many parents how I tested for this sense; they in turn tried the test on each other; it was very humorous to watch them being quite surprised by the results. Remember that these are soft signs that don't mean that much in isolation and we all have some of these signs however if several are present than they are probably significant when these signs are added to the history and the rest of the examination. But remember that these are soft signs they don't mean much on their own, however when there are several or many of these soft signs they do add up added to the history and the observation they add up to the diagnosis. Consider now the example of wanting to cross a busy road; not only do we have to know where we are about to start to cross the road from but we have to know where our body parts are at the time; all this information is crucial if we are to cross the any road successfully. We then have to work out the features of the traffic. We have to work out how far the approaching car is, if we have binocular vision we use that feature, if we don't we have to depend on the noise the car makes to work out how far it is and how fast it is moving. Very quickly we establish if we can get safely across the road before it-the car- gets here; or should we wait until the car drives past us. All the sensory systems, (perhaps some don't have to come into action); but the visual, auditory, vestibular, and the propioception systems integrate so that we can respond appropriately; by the motor behavioral system.

An example of how the sensory systems integrate and compensate for a missing sense can be seen in how blind persons can compensate for the loss of sight. In this example the hearing becomes more acute and so do the other modalities; as a compensation for the loss of one of the senses. Be it because of the loss of the reception organ, or a pathway damage; as it occurs in a stroke; the brain dose and will compensate for sensory losses.

All of these modalities then use the memory sense that will elaborate latter.

A very important aspect of our human brain; is that it has a way to directly communicate between the cortical areas; this does not occur in all other species. Direct communication between areas of the cortex directly to each other allows for a large amount of inputs (information) to be processed. It may be that is the problem with ADHD that they first have to communicate with deeper nuclei and then get back to the cortex; but it is pure conjecture. Add the concentration problems that ADHD children suffer and you can start to imagine how difficult a problem, processing sensory information can become for the child with ADHD.

CHAPTER NINETEEN

—————————⟫•⟪—————————

If we don't keep supporting children that have problems they can end up having a poor self esteem which can affect their whole life. Self-esteem suffers badly when children have these problems; the children themselves do know that they have these troubles and (as a result) perform not as well as their peers that don't have the problems. Take the child with coordination problems and their sporting ability or the child with learning problems and their school result and so on. It is very difficult to keep them positive in the face of their continued failures. We often can make their self esteem worse by pointing out to them their problems (that they are painfully aware off).

Memory problems present a further problem. We often meet people that we have been introduced to before but we can't recall their names at the time we meet them again. How do we feel when we can't recall their names? This is just a very common simple example when memory or recall presents a problem to us. So how bad does a child feel when they can't read or recall the alphabet or the solution to their maths problems and all their friends laugh at them?

Another feature of memory that can be adversely affect many ADHD children is reversals; I have that problem still; I do reverse of numbers so it causes me to spend a lot of extra money on phone calls. How does a child cope with difficulties of memory?

Children with bad memory do wish for good memory not even photographic memories; we meet people that are gifted with photographic memories; how we wish we were like that!

Treating a child for ADHD; that is for their hyperactivity, poor concentration, heightened distractibility and probably their other problems like perceptual problems sometimes gets a bonus of helping them with their behaviour problem. Some children have memory problems too; many times these children just have to learn ways to cope with their poor memories. In the mean time we have to be very understanding and accepting and not fall in the trap of making it worse by expecting that they get over it: or over doctoring them in the efforts to find a solution to their "problem" thus making it very obvious that they do have a problem and we want it fixed. Let me relate to a very interesting experience that I had with a person that had a photographic memory. During my residency; I had colleges of a different race; that was very gifted with a wonderful memory. However he could not apply his wonderful skill. When I was confronted with a medical problem, I would ask him what does the textbook state in relation to this problem. He would tell me, word for word, what the text book stated. It was another matter, when it came to the applying the information. I would then ask him then to tell me exactly what the book states that we should do. He would tell me exactly what it did stated to do. I would ask him then what it is that we must do. He would then reply "I don't know". I would know exactly what to do! As he had just told me what the text book had instructed that we should do; when confronted with such a medical problem. We made a perfect team. He has an excellent memory but he could not apply it; he told me what the text book said that we should do and then I applied the advice.

We are truly unique and so different in our strengths and weakness that we must cherish our differences. Our society is so education obsessed that so often our expectations result in the expectation that every child is academically successful. So for the child that is not academic because often they have many problems; which often include learning problems complicated by bad memory; end up with terrible self esteem and often behaviours problems (conduct disorders). The child feels that they are less valuable, less acceptable, rejected by peers and maybe parents too etc.; is it any wonder that it often results in damage to their self esteem.

I will now return to the assessment; the behaviour is mostly what concerns the teachers, parents, councillors and whoever referred the child. It is not the main aim of treatment so it requires a careful explanation that; we will help with hyper activity, attention and / or distractibility and many other perceptual problems; the result of the treatment is that often we may get a bonus that results in an improvement in their child's behaviours; but it and it will often take time to get the improvements in their behaviours. It is very important to clearly explain this expectation differences. The parent's negative response added to the child's failures; results in exaggerating the child's already poor self-esteem. It is just as important to explain the child really can't help having the problems, they would rather not have them but they do have them. Conduct disorders often do result from untreated ADD so we have to explain that not just medication; but management advice for the whole family will require further interventions. In some cases, parental expectations of learning achievement are not met after the treatment is commenced; it is again important to reset their expectations; to again explain that their child may had so many problems that it will probably take time for the child to catch up with their age group. It is as important not to make the child's self esteem worse by yelling at them because our frustration and of their problems and difficulties. What example are we giving them? Our yelling and frustration in turn often in the child's negativity, and the subsequent conduct and behaviour problems. Over "doctoring"; and seeing many medical specialist, paramedical and alternative medical professionals; does further add to the child's poor self- esteem; especially if they only reinforce by the diagnosis they confirm that the child does have a problem but an effective treatment is not given. The child realizes that the parent just want their problem not to be there; it is usually true that the parent just wants to help the child with their problems; it may not be the parent's intension that they are frustrated because of the problems that the child faces; but the child can misinterpret it in the way that the child is not as desirable (and wanted). Some the parents did not realize or denied their child's had problems; they may have aggravated the problems; by not helping and seeking help for their child; so by not helping they inadvertently caused more damage to the child's self worth-- child's self- esteem. There may be an upside to not labelling the child as different; however it would be better to help the child with their problems than just to leave them to their own devices.

It is important to adequately attend to all the aspects of the child's problems.

CHAPTER TWENTY

I will tell you of a real happening with one of my children. He was born prematurely was constantly vomiting; I have talked of his early life in New Guinea. He started school at the age of five; he was having so much trouble at school that when my wife would pick him up after school; she would have to sit him down in the gutter; she would then feed him lollies so that he would settle enough to get him into the car. By the way we have several controls for our blood sugar in our bodies; so the common belief that sugar is the cause of hyperactivity is based on very poor factual information. I arranged for my child to see an Education School Guidance Officer. When my wife took him to see the Guidance Officer she rang me with so many complaints. One complaint was that he asked her why she helped him so much. She did reply that if she did not she would never get him ready to go anywhere, including school. She was adamant that she would never go back to see him. He must not have been too tactful with his questions on that day. Anyway I did have a lot of faith in him; as he was up to date with ADHD so I managed to convince her to go back. When she went back to see him; straight away his attitude was completely different. He told her to immediately take the child away from that school because amongst other things he told her that the class teacher has a slight accent and that this did complicate his (school) problems. He had already arranged for a special infant mistress to take him into to her school class to help him. She had a special skill in helping kids with ADHD.

He did have ear infections after ear infections. Before his ears were treated; he would often have pus running down his face but he would rarely complain of an ear ache. I suppose it was because his ear drums had burst. She knew that his ears were bad because his behaviour was worse than usual at those times. She would check out if his ears were bad by whispered behind him 'do you want a lolly', if he did not answer her, she knew that his hearing was bad. We to take him to an ENT surgeon; he admitted him to hospital and drained his ears and inserted grommets into his ear drums. One day my wife was called by his grade five teacher. Evelyn and I thought "what now". When she saw the teacher he told her he just wanted to tell her that he had congratulated our child because he went through a whole period without dropping his pencil. He was a wonderful teacher; he would just stand beside our child and place his hand gently on his shoulder until the task was completed. It just goes to show how management is so important and that how a calm persistence works. (At that time condition had not been described; neither had an effective treatment been described for the condition). Our boy is now an adult and a computer consultant; he is running his own business. It does sound like I am really proud of him; and all that my wife has achieved; I am very proud of all of my children with good reason. In grade 11 he was allotted to a class to do ordinary mathematics. Supposedly there was not enough room in the class for advanced math's, so he carried his desk to the advanced math's class asked that teacher if he could stay there. When that teacher said he could, he propped himself there for the rest of the year. He eventually completed a Degree in Business and

Computing at QUT, and later, a degree in adult education. He achieved being a senior lecturer and the head of the information technology department at the Sunshine Coast University. He is one of the few who has achieved Microsoft Gold accreditation. My youngest son is a people's person and was a high earning sales person. Many years later my youngest son is very proud of his brother so he went to the maths coordinator that is still at my older son's school and told him proudly, "you know my brother that you allotted to ordinary maths is a University lecture,". Then he cheekily asked him, "are you still only teaching high school?"

When he stated with his course in business and computing at QUT; back then there was only DOS; my wife asked him do you think there is any future in that industry and will you get a job? It really sounds funny now. All of my other children also have problems with attention, distractibility, short term memory and learning problems. My middle son is more manually inclined and not as academic. He is an A grade mechanic; in most cases he only needs to have a description, even on the telephone what is the trouble with the vehicle; to work out how to fix the problem with the car. He is truly gifted as a mechanic but he still sufferers with poor self-esteem; he did have learning problems and he does not value his achievements because they are not as academic as his brother. The school made it worse in the earlier years because they would say to him" why are you not doing well your father is a doctor your older brother and your sister do really well so why don't you?" A great teacher in his grade 11 supported his great manual skills and partly repaired his poor self-esteem.' He kept on congratulating and honouring his achievements. Both my girls have achieved degrees.

My eldest daughter has a masters teaching in early childhood and a degree in computing. My youngest daughter has a degree in economics she works for a bank and earns good money. All of the families have symptoms and signs consistent with ADD; both their parents have symptoms and signs consistent with ADHD so how could they miss out? (See how important genetic factors are). Neither we nor our children have had medication. The problems were not described and so treatments were not available back then. We and their teachers did manage our children well as their achievements indicate. Infant and children are yet to develop further so supposedly you cannot make such a diagnosis of ADHD before the child is 5 or 6. I do different in this area from the traditional view in that ADHD can be seen from an early age some times. Some mothers do report that their child was different from an early stage. Most mothers, do have a special feel for their children so they do recognizes if their child has the signs of hyperactivity, poor concentration and some of the other signs of ADHD that are present from an early stage. Mothers may report that their child was very different right from the start. Their report is even more useful if he child's mother has other children that she can compare this child with. So I do differ from my colleges in that early diagnosis is possible. I do believe that, in most cases medication is not necessarily, but they and the family should receive appropriate, management advice including counseling of the parent and family therapy if required as these measures can prevent further future problems developing later. "What is normal"?

As a student, I had to write an assignment on exactly that very topic. After several pages of writing, I arrived at the conclusion that there was so many ways to look at the concept; that it was very much the way you wish to define normal. In any case, I would like you to consider the concept that Attention Deficit Disorder is probably a <u>variant of normal.</u> Perhaps it is a <u>developmental problem.</u> In our **society**; that does value education so much, ADHD is seen as such a problem because of the many learning and memory problems. 'Children' are expected to stay at school well into their mature ages, sometime to age19 or longer. If they want to go to University or to further their education they stay at "school" even longer. It suites some people but not others. If you are not made that way (academically) it is horrible. In this age, we can help ADHD. There is something that we can do for ADHD. Treatment options are available to enable our children to deal with the demands of our **society**. Academic school results are very much valued. Manual skills are not valued as much, even though they are extremely important. Adolescents are expected to stay at school until they are young men; their hormones and development results in the natural attraction to the opposite gender and so they are ready to start manhood. But they are expected to stay at school and concentrate on academic issues. Nature dictates that boys find girls interesting and girls find boys very attractive, so is it any wonder that some young men and women are no longer interested in school work. In co-educational schools, you can observe why the opposite gender becomes so interesting and distracting. In traditional schools, some of the the pupils find it much more interesting to contemplate and discuss the week-end activities rather than try to concentrate on the "boring" stuff such as school work. The boys probably start looking toward their sexual needs, the girl look to finding a potential partner. Children that started school early or that started with problems like ADHD or Asperger's most probably still have not caught up physically or emotionally to their peers. The boys don't consider them desirably in the sports arena etc. because their ability, coordination, maturity or other problems. Girls seem to mature earlier; the girls find them so immature; are often small; so they less attractive because they are younger and probably less able at sporting activities. What's more girls can be very derogatory at this age. So overall that is a further blow to their self- esteem of ADHD children. In many societies; that are considered primitive (backwards), adolescents move out of the family home as soon as they reach adolescence and begin their adult life. But in our society they are still expected to stay at school and therefore in the family home.. It is lucky that we can help children to cope with the demand of our society. A tribe in Africa was recently discovered and studied; almost all the population of that village has features that are consistent with the diagnosis of ADHD. Their community consists of mainly shepherds, so in their community ADHD is considered an advantage. The activity they seem to possess stands them in good stead. In Darwin's theory we develop feature that allow us to better survive in our society. Is ADHD a feature for the survival of the fittest in that society? So is ADHD a normal variant? Are we interfering in the normal development in 'our' society? What an interesting question! Again I would like you to consider this thought, and look at ADD or ADHD as variant of normal. In our society and at this time ADHD does present us with a problem. Thank goodness that there is an effectively treatment has been identified for ADHD and (Aspergius) so that a child can reach their potential in our society. Again I want to repeat that our society is a complicated society and it values academic education so much.

Children with these problems are often ridiculed or rejected by their friends, their peers, their teachers and sometimes by our very own friends. Is it any wonder that so many often have a lifelong poor self-esteem?

They can't help it. It is reasonable, to deprive them of effective treatment, and management advise. I would go as far as to say it is negligent to deprive them of effective treatment or to delay further their effective treatment and management. If we neglect to provide adequate treatment for our child's medical condition is it not negligent and punishable by law; so why is ADHD or Asperger's different? I can understand the advice that makes parents so nervous; that they stop effective treatments because of dramatic reports by unprofessional reporting in the media of the very rare side effects of effective medications. Any treatment involves possible side effects they must be carefully monitored; so that these side effects are less of a problem. I feel so strongly (you can see how emotive I get) for the children are deprived of effective treatment' or their treatment is interrupted by these dramatic reports. It is the child that misses out; hopefully it is only for a time but even then it can have long term consequences.

One such report that was printed in the Courier Mail some years ago, in infuriated me so much that I consulted a solicitor to see if I could sue the newspaper for the report. It was a whole lift out section of several pages. It only had two part columns from traditional practitioners (that do work in this area). I am sure that they were asked leading questions because their comment seemed to support the idea that these mediations had the side effect. That the whole article was about the terrible side effects; of course that is a known side effect; it is extremely rare and careful monitoring of the patient condition is essen ADHD tial. The proponents that were reported in this article are more interested in their ineffective treatments and their pockets than the children! In any case, because of the freedom of the press, the solicitor advised me that it would be futile try and sue the paper. I ask you is it responsible reporting when it hurt our children. At another time a report by a famous paediatrician caused several parents to stop their child's medication; luckily the medication can be stopped suddenly. Incidentally he later retracted his earlier comments. Many of the parents that had stopped their child's medication because of his first article did return later, asking that the child start treatment again. Unfortunately it is the child that did missed out for a while because of that report. Perhaps the report was well meaning, but it was ill considered.

Often a medical diagnosis can be used as a label. The name of a diagnosis is the so that practitioners can talk to each other; and so that they do understand the condition that they are talking about; they can then prescribe appropriate management and treatments for our society that apply; that they have been found after expensive and painstaking research to work. The label can be used in ways that it was not meant to be used in; The label can be used by children themselves as an excuse for their bad behaviour, as a taunt to torture a child further, an excuse for our yelling due to our frustration and to blame the child, even when it is not their fault and by parents when they don't control the child. One of my children that had the learning problem; the school tried to help by getting him to attend the remedial classes; he refused to attend those classes because he told us that his peers called the remedial class the "veggie class"

I have told you of the really "funny" experience that I had when I was a resident at Geelong hospital. Regularly in the mornings, this particular child would present to casualty with a multitude of symptoms. Examination was always negative. So when I told him he could go to school he would say "you know I am mentally retired", He was trying to use a label he had heard. Sometimes it does result in, especially the adolescent child, rejecting the diagnosis and refusing the treatment as a result of not wanting to be taunted by their peers. You can understand children not wanting to be called 'Veggies' by their peers when they get called to the office for their medications or to go to the special education unit. In no way does it mean that ADD corresponds to retardation. Some parents are very understanding because of this problem; they try the ineffective treatments in the hope that they will work. Many a time even the patients and the parent come to realize that they need the effective treatment. Sometimes parents just don't want to accept that there is something 'wrong' with their child; one or both parents may have had a similar problem themselves; they use any excuse not to use appropriate medication. Some parents use the excuse that they have read some report on the internet or seen a report on the media or a good friend; has told them of some treatment that works so well; so they do try it because it suits them so well. They seem to prefer to try the ineffective treatments alternatives (usually they are more expensive).But it is their child that misses out Because ADHD is quite a common enough problem in our society; many people come up with alternative treatments many are then publicized by the media or the internet. Some parents are initially are convinced that some alternative treatment worked well for their child. Mind you there is such a thing as the placebo effect and the more expensive a treatment is the more likely the placebo effect works; initially at least. Later I will discuss many of these ineffective alternative treatments; some of these include such things like the diet, the A2 milk, colored glasses, fish oil, pycnogenol and the list goes on and on.

Eventually most parents do realize that the traditional medicine treatment is the only one that is effective. I have a real concern that while parents are confused and consider their options it is the children that are missing out on effective treatments. They go on failing because of their learning problems so they have to put up with rejection from peers, and even from you own so called friends; and so on it goes! Sometimes a parent has had, or still has similar problems (and had to deal with them without appropriate help); so they don't accept that their child will do better with medication. I do have some parents in my practice that say "I did ok so there is need for medication;. My response would be "you most likely could have done so much better had this condition been described and you were treated effectively." It has sometimes worked especially with that they recognize the difficulties they had faced and then they do accept the treatment for their child. I can understand that on one hand a parent did get on without treatment in the; (but the correct treatment was not yet available), and the other hand dramatic reports appear in the press or media casting great doubt on the treatment; these reports dramatically project the idea that medication is not good and they emphasis the possible side effect. Is it any wonder that concerned parents have so many apprehensions about medication treatments? Side effects are rare, but they do occur, so the patients have to be watched carefully and followed up closely. The packet insert with any medication' by law include product information that including any possible side effects. They are a good thing, however they are often what I call 'scare sheet' as they are very scary especially for the anxious patient or parents. As they seem to gets all the possible side effects.

You can see how emotive I do get when because of misreporting, it only results in great unnecessary anxiety and it results that some children have to and do unnecessarily suffer. Unfortunately, when a parent denies that there is a problem; in spite of explaining and demonstrating the problem to them and they still deny the problem: or worse they blame the other parent for not controlling the child properly; they often refuse help for their child. It is the child that misses out when a parent refuses to have treatment for whatever the reason. I repeat it does feel negligent; if for any reason the parent refuses to give their child effective treatment.

CHAPTER TWENTY-ONE

———— ⟫·⟪ ————

The brain is an organ, but it actually has many centres. It controls so many functions. Yet when such a complex organ as the brain has a problem, some people find that treatment is difficult to accept. If one has diabetes, usually, one accepts that treatment is essential. Many people, and so called experts, have a lot of difficulty accepting that brain condition that are not physical need treatment as any other sickness does It is probably that the brain is only partially understood, and that people have the left over concept that treatment of emotional problems is compared to being mad. The treatment of neurological (physical) problems seems to be more easily accepted.

Now for a very funny diversions; I have an 17th century text of medical conditions and their treatment that is very funny in parts; one part describes the treatment for depression at that time; it involved being tied by the ankles and dipped in a vat of cold water alternating with dipping you into hot water. If you were not depressed after that early shock treatment you would probably be worse. I do want to tell you of a very funny diagnosis of that time; there is a picture of a healthy well built young man; next to it there is a picture of a shrivelled up old man; the caption under the picture reads that is the result of masturbation! The brain has centres to deal with sensory inputs. The olfactory centre in our species is much smaller than it is in some other species like canines where it is much bigger for smell because dogs use their smell sense extensively. In humans that area of the brain has been taken over for the functions of emotions, sexual drives, memories and anger. In a condition called temporal epilepsy patients suffering this condition they may experience episodes of unprovoked anger. This condition is important to exclude in children that presents because of explosive temper. It may need extensive investigation, often requiring a sleep EEG (electroencephalogram). This is usually done after consultation with a neurologist experienced with children. In other cases the patient may experiences feeling of having been to a place that they have not been to before; they are called déjà vu experiences; some others patient experience strange smells. One adult patient that I have seen calls these her Wobblies. Nobody else can see her experiencing them. The gustatory (taste) sense is interesting, e.g. the parents' of children suffering with ADD often report various likes by their children such as sour plums or obsession with sweet things, like sugar. I don't know whether this is a feature of taste malfunction or more of their obsessions. Tactile sense includes pain, soft touch, vibration and temperature sense. The visual sense is the sense of sight. The reception area is at the back of the brain. The eyes receive the light then they transmitted by the optic nerves to the back of the brain. The auditory centres use the ears as receptors. The Speech areas are located in the dominant lobe of the brain and the auditory areas are closely related to them. The vestibular organs are located in the middle ear. The balance system connections are very complicated as several nuclei are involved some are in the cerebellum some are in the pons and so on. The propioception senses are recorded and perceived in the brain. I intend to elaborate more about these senses later

CHAPTER TWENTY-TWO

I refer you to the diagram in chapter twenty of the model that I proposed to better understand ADHD. The model comparers our brain to a large main frame computer. The hereditary factors determine the hardware; it does so by way of the DNA that we inherit. It also has a program that determines the steps that we should go through to amass the information that we collect and store during our life. This is the software as it were. Then the information that we collect during our life is like then programming that we undertake. Then our reactions to stimuli can be thought of as behaviour in its broadest sense. These can be the motor responses, communication and or just thoughts. The main frame computer consists of two sides side by side as it were. One side deals with emotional material while the other side deals with rational inputs. The two sides can communicate and change previous programming but it does require a lot of effort. The output behaviour results from the balance of the inputs to the two sides. The both sides are programmed according to a preset age dependent format. This programming can be adjusted as times goes by, however it is much more difficult but it can happen. For example counselling when we are adults can slowly adjust for experiences in childhood etc. This programming takes place in some form of age order. This order is not completely fixed so some parts take place while some other stage is being completed. There are the seven of inputs our sensory pathways channels, the keyboard as it were. We respond by thoughts, speech and other motor responses.

The seven input channels that provide us with the sensory information. These are the **Gustatory** (taste) **Olfactory** (smell) **Tactile** (feeling system) (of bodies sensations, with the four division, namely soft touch, pain, temperature and vibration senses). **Visual** (sight) **Auditory** (hearing) **Vestibular** (balance sense), **Propiosensory** (body information), The response channels are the **Motor responses,** either speech or motor or though response. These are the broad behavioural responses to stimuli. The unique feature of the human being's brain is the ability to communicate directly from the cortical areas of the brain to another part of the cortical areas without first going to the deeper areas (thalamus). In primitive species the communication has to goes first to thalamus from the cortex and then back to the relevant area of cerebral cortex. Before the sensory input channels have been programmed the infant communicates with its mother by what is called the **General sensor Mechanism.** It was an Australian child psychiatrist by the name of Michael Rutherford that first described this mechanism. During the first few weeks of a child's life, before the sensory pathways have been programmed, the child communicates with their mother by way of this General Sensor Mechanism. You can observe the comfort that mother's cuddles provide. Incidentally you can observe how mother's tension is also conveyed. Take the example of a young inexperienced mother is trying to comfort her distraught infant with no success. Grandmother tells her "Give me the child and I will show you how it is done". The child settles down quickly. Was it the grandmother's technique? No it was her confidence. The infant responded to her calmness. It does serve to make the already uptight mother feel bad; she then thinks that she was doing it all wrong but in fact it was her uptightness. Her mother or mother in law probably made it worse when they told her that she did not know how to care for her baby as she is so inexperienced. Another very interesting is feature of the General Sensor Mechanism is best demonstrated by the following example; a lady that grew up in an abusive family usually marries an abusive or controlling husband. Interestingly, the love for our parents occurs during the time that the General Sensor Mechanism is the only sense that is operating. Even though in reason, the girl in this example may hate her father because of the abuse to herself, or witnessing the abuse her mother tolerates, she usually ends up choosing a partner with a similar personality as her father's. Boys may end up being abusers, in spite of hating abuse that they have experience or witnessed. It is often said most girls marry men with similar personalities as their 'father' or boys marry women with similar personalities as their 'mothers'. How often do we see children taking up the occupation that is similar or the same as their parents? Even after a divorce and extensive counselling, people end up marring for a second or third time a partner with similar qualities to their first partner that they loved and married. The ability to 'feel' because of the General Sensor Mechanism does persist, however it is over shadowed by the more specific systems. I am sure you can relate to this feature, you can recall meeting a person and you immediately love or hate that person. You try to figure out why that is. Does it remind you of somebody you knew? Sometimes it does but most times you can't figure out why. This is a good example that the general sensory mechanism still operates.

All of the input channels integrate. If one input channel is damaged or inoperative then another channel seems become more sensitive to replace the damaged channel. A typical example is that of a blind person's hearing seems to become more acute if the visual pathway does not work.

There is one main frame computer that consists of two sides that are side by side. These sides communicate with each other to some extent. One side deals with the concrete inputs while, the other side deals with the emotional inputs. Imagine now a beam balance that decides the balance of emotional input that goes into the computer and the input that goes into the rational side of the computer. Another way to say this is the balance between the emotional input and the concrete input is decided by beam balance angle. The amount of input that goes into each sides of the computer is decided by the beam balance position. If the beam balance is tilted towards the emotional side then the rational input is greater than the emotional input. So the reaction by the behaviour is more emotional. If it is tilted the other way then the emotional input would be greater and the output behaviour would reflect that. You can observe the emotional over reactions of ADHD children, especially when they are tired or hungry. Another feature that I designed was that the beam balance mechanism can be sticky and does not change very easily so it is more often tilted so the input is more emotional and hence so is the output. A child with ADHD often reacts impulsively and then thinks of the consequences of its actions. This is because they do respond emotionally, according to the emotional input and not necessarily rationally. You have probably seen a funny bumper car sticker that reads 'put your brain into gear before you open your mouth'. You can think of many examples of an ADHD child reacting from emotions rather than reacting rationally. I will talk later how the ADD treatment stimulates the control (rational) part of the brain after they impulsively react. The beam balance can be affected by so many factors, as I said it can be sticky. The behavioural responses depend on this balance and at the age of the child. The output or behaviour channels allow us to respond to this input balance. These responses rely on previous information that was learnt during the developmental stages that I will now describe.

The computers have a predetermined order that the need to be programmed in. This is according to age of the child and his or her development. All the stages are very important as you will see as we go along. In the first 18 months the child has to program its input channels. It is believed that if a part of this stage is missed it can and does have an effect on latter perceptual developments. As an example; if a stage is missed, as is seen with infants that miss the crawling stage because their mother has them in a "walker' most of the child's infancy, that is until the child starts walking (horizontally) thus walking without experiencing the crawling stage. Another example of this stage is-your child is happy to see you and smiles at you when you come home from work. However, on the next occasion; you come home still wearing your hat, the young child does not recognize you worse he or she start crying till you take off your hat and then you are recognized. Later in their development, the child will no longer have this problem. I do personally relate to a similar experience; when I first went to Papua New Guinea I could not tell one native from another. As I got to know them I could recognize them individually, and by name. At first we do learn to recognize things by their main features, later we learn to look at more details. Now; I will return to this predetermined developmental stage. During this stage the child gets as much information as it can about his/her sense; The child plays with mother's pots and pans, it imitates what it sees, it may play with cold water on a cold day, even though mother tell him/her to stop, but the child just wants to experience the water. The child is into everything it can, it wants to experience its senses and what they can provide his/her about the environment. After the first 18 months, the child is ready to control what it has learnt .So now comes the first "'no" stage.

We can call this the terrible two's.

During this stage of the development, the word 'no' is often heard. We hear; 'no' for the sake of 'no' It is an important stage it is the first control stage as the child learns to control what the child has learnt. It is important not to over or under control the child. The child says 'no' for the sake of controlling the experiences it has collected. For example, mother tells him to stop playing with the cold water or they will get a cold. The child will often reply 'no' I won't stop.

The child moves on to the friendly '3's'. This is again a very important stage. The child learns how to handle people. Obviously the first contact the child has is with the family. I often give the example of this stage where the child is at grandmother's place; the child says "I love you grandma" then in the same breath says 'where do you keep the choc grandma?'" It is very important to know how to handle people. A common saying goes like so "it is not what you know but who you know. I add it is how well you do know you know them.

The <u>bossy '4's'</u> is the next stage. These stages do go in order but the next stage can proceed while the previous stage is being completed. I often quote an example that many parent can identify with; it goes like so; at two the child say no, I won't stop playing with the cold water, but they are easy to convince. At 4 year old the child says no and means it; another typical example is that when the child is told to go and have a bath (or shower) they reply. 'No no no". When they say no they mean it. This is another important control stage. The parental response is very important with any children but even more so with ADD. Again too much control can be potentially damaging. If the parent is too tolerant the child gets away with it and learns to defy next time. If, on the other hand, the parent is too strict and controlling, the child does not learn to stand up for itself and may become too compliant or they become rebellious; the child can go either way; they can start being very (too) compliant but as they come into adolescence they can become rebellious; not just to the parents but to authority too. I firmly believe it is essential for the child to have fair limits. The balance is very important. Like everything in life too much of anything or not enough of anything results in a bad thing. It is like it is with food" too much food and a person gets fat and it is not healthy; not enough nutrition and the result are equally unhealthy.

<u>5 year old</u> stage I call the 'why' stage. The child constantly says why to everything. When he asks the father a "how was I born" the farther think how will I explain to the child all the ins and outs of their creation so he says typically "go and ask your mother". The mother; knowing her child well, tells the child you were delivered at the Royal Brisbane Hospital! The child goes away happily and resumes playing.

The 6 & 7 year old; the child progresses to organizing and controlling the information that they have collected. During this stage they may ask a question and if your answer is not correct they will consult an encyclopaedia. Or in these days it probably will be the internet. Then they will come back to us and point out how we were wrong. A beautiful advertisement for the Big Pond internet provider; that I really like demonstrated this point. A child asks his father a simple question "why was the great wall of China built?' The father thinks for a second then he replied :it was built to keep the rabbits out!" I am sure that child would look up encyclopaedia or in this day the internet, and point out to his father it was not built to keep rabbits out.

At 7, 8 or 9 the next thing that we do have to learn about is that we have to belong and deal with groups. The child learns to belong to their group. A typical request by your child may be; all the children at my school have Reeboks (shoes). So please get me a pair 'I don't want to be the odd one out". "If you are a boy, girls are yuck. They even have girl germs. If your child is a girl boys are just naughty. Our world does consist of groups of people so it is important to learn about groups, to learn what group we want to belong to; what people in our group we want to aspire to be like; and what are groups that we want to (need) avoid, We also learn such things as loyalty to 'our' group

The 9 to 13 year age group. By the passing of a few years the child moves on to the next stage. Usually their hormones are starting to build up in their systems. They start to look after their appearance, they even shower without being asked and they use deodorant. They spend hours doing their hair in front of the mirror for hours to make sure their hair is just right; if your child is a boy that particular girl does not have girl germs..

From <u>13 to 19 </u>years of age they then move onto learning about ideals. I say that if you want to find a fault with anything just ask a typical teenager. I am sure that that they will tell you where you are wrong. The child is now a young adult and they do learn what is correct and what is wrong. They learn by the examples that their parents live by.

<u>19 to 25.</u> In a few more years they are quite surprised how quickly their parents have learned the exception to the rules. Do you tell the police where your brother is if they are looking for him for a minor misdoing? During this stage they learn that in complex situations there is not a simple answer.

<u>25 to 40.</u> Our development is almost complete as far as our personal needs are concerned. So after choosing a partner we move onto raising our family. The next generation then usually begins. I again repeat that children learn better by example rather than just words so good example is so important.

<u>40 to 60.</u> We then move on and join community groups as the next generation of children grow up. We often take on voluntary work if our-health is o.k. We watch our children raise their children, we are proud of their achievement and we prepare for our retirement.

The <u>age of 60</u> goes on to completion of life's travel. During retirement parents baby sit, they often travel, and they join the "ski" club – "Spend your Kids" inheritance. Often they watch their children make the same mistakes as they did and they prepare for their funeral and a celebration of their life. ".

I did find that a lot of parent could identify with the stages that I described.

So in summary, we learn our sensory inputs then we learn to control them; we then move to learn the next thing in our world- people! We have to learn how to deal with people and then how to manage them, not to be overrun by them. Next in our world is information, so again we first learn how to get information and then how to use it. Our world is large and so for most of us we have to deal with groups as this is a team world. We learn how to belong to a group and then how to handle different groups. Our world has ideals and moral codes so our program includes a stage when we go learn to deal with these. There are exceptions to rules so we have to learn to handle these exceptions. Now we are ready to start the circle again and bring up the next generation. The older generation moves on to watching on (as grandparents). Many seniors take on community responsibilities. They often baby sit for their children when they can.

 These progressive stages are basically fixed, however as I have said the rate in which they are completed is variable. It is possible to move on to the next stage while still finishing the previous one.

It takes a lot of therapy to change our automatic feelings that we learned both by education and the witnessing (modelling). We, do have a feedback system as humans, however it is difficult to alter what we originally learnt as a child.

CHAPTER TWENTY-THREE

———◆))‧((◆———

I have been lecturing to group of fathers with a movement called, Fathers Caring for Kids since its foundation; I consider that this group is so important. I wish to present the lecture I gave to the groups, and to present you the information that I collected from this groups. I will start to talk of the topic of my presentation and then I will go on and talk about some of the issues that many of the groups brought up. I presented the introductory lecture; the topic of which was the "Importance of modelling." I began my presentation using the idea of a business plan. I started by exploring what qualities that the fathers wanted for their children; all the groups of father did want much the same qualities for their children. I would then explore how they would go about obtain these qualities in their children. I expect that we all want much the same for our next generation; our children. I'd proceed asking each of the fathers one quality they desired for their children to have; as I went around and asked each farther what qualities they wanted for their child I would write them down on a white board. I would underline this quality that the individual fathers' emphasized. I found that the quality of discipline was repeated so often. All the groups felt that the quality of the child had been brought up to respect discipline is of the utmost importance. They felt that they have to ensure that the child has learnt the value of discipline. They have to be brought with discipline (limits), so that the child grows up correctly. The child has to learn the value of self-discipline too. Many groups of fathers did bring up that is was now a day a very difficult the job to be a parent because of so many outside influenced; like the availability of drugs and this technological era. They all seem to desire much the same qualities for their children. The qualities that they desired their children to obtain were-

Discipline Happiness seems to be to be every ones desire. Self-esteem (but not arrogance). Respect for others, including family, friends, society and authority as well as themselves. Good ability to communicate and relate well (it is often who you know and not what you know and how well you get on with them).

Successful (at what they choose to do!). Honesty and Fairness to others. Good Moral Standards and Values. Respect for Alcohol, and Drugs. They wanted their children to avoid addictions. E.G. gambling and drugs. (Cigarettes were brought up sometimes I will start with the topic of discipline; it was always very emotive, and all the groups always wanted to talk about this topic at great length.

I found that I would always have to start with a discussion about the difference between punishment and discipline as there seem that a problem does exist in this area. Discipline or limit setting is for the child's benefit and not to relieve our frustration; (or it does become punishment) A lot of the fathers did experienced punishment. So they believe that punishment is actually discipline. Consistent limit setting is of the utmost importance bringing up any child; it is especially important with children that suffer with ADD and ADHD; so disciple has to set limits clearly; it has to be discipline and not punishment; it has to be fair, not belittling and in no way aggressive. I would ask the groups to recall their own experiences. According to my definition they would invariably agree that they were actually punished. However they often pointed out that it did not do them any harm and that it did serve them well; it was an important learning experience to know their boundaries. They would emphasis that discipline is very important (even if it is punishment and it is harsh), it is better to have clear limit and consequences than not have any at all. They discussed; very emotively; that the present system of "No Physical Punishment" has caused a big problem in our society. It has been an attempt to stop punishment, although it is a good intension, has it gone too far? Have we removed too many limits? We have become too soft, as a society. The children know their rights and quote them to us, but their responsibilities are not emphasized. They could point out many examples of when children do not have limits or consequences they turn out as children and young adults without boundaries. Their behaviour includes alcohol abuse, fighting and lawlessness. I have seen children start drinking at primary school. Alcohol fuels their fights, and they even go looking for fights. They said that this generation is facing a problem today because discipline has been eroded. That today's social problems are a result of very poor discipline or even none existent discipline. Schools do not have any the power to administer consequences for bad behaviour. The schools today end up suspending (or expelling) a child for repeated misbehaviours; they write a letter to the child's parents and expect them to follow through with the suspension. That is often useless as some children learn to use this system for their benefit – I will talk more about this later. In their day, and their parent's day, the school did have the tools to administer limits and they did work. Some children have not learned limits yet and the school can teach their pupil limits but they no longer want the responsibility to teach more than it was better in the long run than today's system.

They would often see children that played up at school and ended getting suspended; they would consider it a reward. I agree as I often had it said to me "it is good to have a day off to sleep-in then play with the play station or just play".

Fundamentally the intention is good, school suspensions will only work if the parent supervises the child and ensure that the child does their school work at home, not to play or sleep in. After all is said and done it is the parents' responsibility to see that their child grows up with discipline. In reality some parents don't do their job properly; and in previous generations schools picked the pieces however nobody seems to care about the child. A lot of the father in the many groups brought up that many of parents especially the mothers are too soft and don't stop the children from doing what they want. They also said that some mothers are too eager to believe their child is telling the truth even when the facts don't point that way. I'd often get comments that the mothers are a major part of the problem. Remember that this is a father group that is disillusioned with marriage. They would quote me the example of the child's mother going to school blaming the school and not believing the teacher or headmaster. Many of the different groups repeatedly told me that mothers tell them (the fathers) to make a child behave, but when they try; the mothers get upset and they say that the father did not do it right. It always ends up in argument between the parents; and the child goes to play and gets away with misbehaving. I'd try to point out that there is a special bond between mother and child, and because of this aspect the mother experiences the child's feelings (the General Sensor Mechanism).

Many fathers brought up the topic of bulling. Accepting personal responsibility seems to be going out the window and we are always looking out for somebody else to sort out our problems. They felt it is the result that children are not allowed to fight; if a child tries to stand up to the bully they will often get into trouble themselves for fighting. I point out that ADHD children usually have bad coordination, so they often get a beating if they do try to stand up to a bully, so it is up to the adults to try to stamp out this bulling. In their day they were told by their fathers to stand up for themselves so there was not as much bulling as there is now because the bullies did not get away with that behaviour as they do now. They pointed out that often they did have a friend that would stand up to the bully for them but they too are afraid of getting into trouble for fighting so the bully keep on bulling as they get away with it in our present system. We have so much of a problem now and it is because our present system has created it; it is so bad that you can read that some children have been driven to tragically suicide. They strongly believed that the strap should be brought back to schools. The consensus was that only the headmaster should be allowed to administer it fairly and after obtaining parental consent. If the parents are not willing to give consent but the child's behaviour is totally not acceptable, then the Education Department approval should be obtained. They do grant that it should be used only as a last resort and with the utmost of care. Again and again they bring up that the strap was used when they were at school and it did them no harm and it did teach them respect. They again reiterated that today's system is not working because the school does not have any power so that children don't have any respect for the school, the teacher or the headmaster.

Another group of fathers emphasized that they felt that the present fashion of suspensions does not really work. Some kids even play up to get suspended, it really just punishes the parents and family as one parent often has to stay home from work. So this punishes the whole family as the families income suffers. One parent has to forego the wages for the days of suspension. In these days of tight budgets, it can be a major further stress that will affect the whole family. Again, they emphasized to me that some children like their suspensions, they like not having to do school work and not having to get up early. Perhaps they can even stay up late watching T.V. and on the next day just play. This group of fathers was very emotive when they brought up again how some mothers are too soft; they let the child do as they want and not do as they are told to do. Because that particular group was getting so emotional; I tried to change the subject by talking about the difficulties that result if the parents don't see eye to eye but it did not work. That group returned to the emotive and heated discussion; about how most mothers were part of the problem. Again, remember that the groups of fathers that have separated from their wives. Perhaps it was even because the parents disagreed so much on how to manage the child. If the father tried to make the child as they were told their by their exasperated wives it would only end up in an argument. The child was being very oppositional and did refuse to do as they were told. The mother failed to get a result, so words alone would not work. The child needed a certain amount of force to be controlled. The mother felt the father did not do it as she wanted it done and the farther was too aggressive. As a result a heated argument between the parents followed; the other children were upset and crying so they were sent to their rooms. The parents would end up keeping on arguing so the offending child ended up of the hook; so the focus was no longer on them so they go on to play happily. Some children even get to know the pattern and learn use it. They went on to repeat some of the comment of other groups that mothers are too eager to believe their child is telling the truth even when the facts don't point that way.

They then turn to discuss some of the present problems that result because of the present school admiration. Many schools use a coloured card system to warn children of their misdoings. If that still does not work they then suspend the child from attending school. They say that this may be a reward for many children, but it is a punishment for many working parents. Many stresses result on the whole family because of the suspension or the expulsion. The responsible parent has to make sure the child does his work and often that is up to the mother. Sometimes the child is given work to do at home, but sometimes the work is not given. The child has usually been suspended because they have been rebellious, so mother has little chance of making the child do as they are told. If the father tries to gain control; it often results in an argument and the child is again is of the 'hook' when the parent start to argue. More often than not, the children are left to their own devices and school work is the last thing on their minds. When the child does go back to school, they have missed certain lessons which are important. They may have been given the lesson as homework but did they do it?

There seemed to be a break in the conversation with that particular group so I seized the opportunity to continue with my presentation- the the importance of the father as a role model. I then returned to talk about all the qualities that the fathers wanted and the way to obtain these for their children was by that example teaches much better than words. I proceeded by presenting some personal examples of experiences that the fathers could identify with. One evening as I was late night shopping at Kmart, I heard a woman yelling at her child "Don't you yell at me in that way" I did not hear the child yelling at her mother! Who was yelling? Not the child but the mother was yelling! This is a good example, of the importance of modeling. Do as I say but don't do as I do! Or one can say monkey see monkey do. Example is as a very important teaching tool. I gave them another personal example; on a Sunday morning we often got a knock the front door from two well suited gentlemen they would give us a sermon and then would try to sell us their Watch Tower magazine publication. We did not like to be rude so we would pretend not to be at home and get everyone to be quiet, and wait until they left. On one Sunday at 8.30am the children; some of them teenagers by then; did not want to come with us to church; they offered to look after the younger ones; so we went on our own. We lived in the large two story house in Kallangur (I have described). On our return, the front door was open. We called out to our children, but we did not get any answer. As we did not get a reply so we stated to worry! We went upstairs to look for the children. We could not find the children and then we heard one of our younger children whispering from inside a cupboard; the older ones were telling him to be quite. He whispered 'did they come upstairs?' We were very so relieved that we found them in the cupboard. They were being very quiet in an upstairs bedroom! We asked why they did not answer" they replied "those people" you know those men with their pamphlets knocked on the door, so we all went upstairs and hid in the cupboard until they left"! Mind you they left the front door wide opened all the time! My father lived across the road at the time; he came over to tell the men that there was somebody at home so the men waited for a while, but when nobody came to the open door they left. Again that demonstrated how our children copied what they had seen us do previously. This is a wonderful example of monkey see monkey do!

I asked the group consider some other examples; picture now a father sitting on the couch watching the evening news on the TV; he orders the children to help their mother to set the table! Would it not be much better for the children to see the father actually helping the children to set the table? The children would see how a father should help! They in turn would learn how it is to be like a father like their father; does it serve as the example of how to be a good partner; when it is their turn to be a family man! Did he give them the example of how they should behave when it is their turn to become a father?

Another scenario that I "painted" for the group was that we often wanted a child to back off in an argument, if we want the child to learn backing off should we first give them the example by doing so? Again that goes for apologizing; we must give them the example first. This of course rarely happens!

Another fathers group again brought the fact that the strap was no longer used in school. They pointed out that the discipline in private schools is often better than it is in public schools so many parents try to send their children to private schools because the discipline is much better but they don't use the strap. They again brought up that children are not allowed to fight in schools but they added another important dimension to the discussion. They felt that schools are toothless when it comes to consequences; but worse when children that are not allowed to fight back the children are told to go to a teacher if they are bullied. They tell to me that when they tell their child to go to the teacher to tell them they are being bullied; they are sometimes told not to be such tattle tails. I pointed out that many of the children who are the bullies often have problems themselves so the school staff tries to be understanding to them. I pointed out how hard it can be to be sympathetic to the child that was bullied and also to make allowances for the circumstances of the bully. The courts often have the same dilemma with it comes to sentencing criminals. It can be very difficult but the school teacher's hands are often tied. All the fathers of that group insisted that the bullied child is often disadvantaged; in our society too many allowances and excuses are made for unacceptable behaviours. In the cases of persistent bulling; it would seem that will take some parent to sue the school before something is done to stop this making too allowances for the law breaker. It would seem that in today society that aggression works better than politeness and consideration for others. They again made the point that our society made too many allowances for the law breaker and it starts at schools because respect for authority has been removed!

Another fathers group made the point that so many changes have occurred in our society that is difficult to keep up. The technological advances have resulted in many positive advances. I pointed out the medical advances have resulted in better treatments so that we have greater life expectation; the diagnosis of condition like ADHD has been described; and treatments for conditions like ADHD etc, are now possible; parenting styles have changed so they have realized that physical punishment is better avoided.

They stated that perhaps it has gone too far because the importance of limit setting and discipline may be have been eroded so that some children quote their rights and don't respect their elders let alone their peers, they may start drinking or taking drugs from a young age, drugs which cause more problems are now easily available. We only had alcohol and cigarettes in our day. As a result of drug abuse children become more aggressive and get into more fights. Education has changed so much that it is difficult nowadays to try to explain to children the way that we solved problems and to be told 'that is not how we do it' (now), information is readily available, by the press, radio, television, the internet provide us with dramatic reports (often) that it is difficult to know what is correct.

Another of the group of fathers discussed that many of children come from an abusive households. They are used to violence and they are often abusive themselves. They are the peers of our children and they provide our impressionable children with bad examples. They are often bullies and can tell lies with a straight face. In the past generation people believed that if you were in an unsatisfactory relationship, which is non loving or worse, abusive- the parents should stay together and wait until the children grew up before they separated. We know now that the sooner a child stops being or witnessing abuse the better. Either the children are abused themselves; either sexually or physically, or they witness their mothers being verbally or physically abused. When a child is from an abusive environment they learn from the example. During our early life, before we get to the age of reason at about 6 or 7 years old, we do have emotions however and because we love our parents even though we in reason we may not like what they do. None the less, when kids grow to identifying with the parent they love even though they do not like what they go through the boys end up like their fathers and the girls end up similar to their mother. They may be loving and supporting, or controlling and or aggressive as the case may be! That group made a very important point that our older children are influenced by their friends and we have less influence as they grow up. I did emphasis that our modelling when they are young is very important and the children choose peers with similar valued that they saw when they were young. I had been in practice long enough to see children grow up and witness abuse or be abused themselves. Often the girls hated the situation of being abused or watching their mother being abused but they end up finding and loving an abusive, or at best a controlling partner. Provided that they don't stay in the relationship too long; to end up having all their self esteem totally destroyed. If they finally manage to get out of the abusive relationship, but they often end up with another partner with similar personality; abusive or controlling. They may be able do manage to change what I call the "cycle" but it does take extensive support and counselling to affect a change; I have seen it happen.

The boys that grow up in an abusive household often grow to hate what they experienced, nevertheless they often become the abusive or at best 'control freak' husbands. I really don't know why it is that a few children break this cycle of abuse'. Perhaps it is because a favored child usually finds it very difficult to change, but a rejected child hates the situation so much that they end up changing the cycle; not following the pattern that they experienced. I can give you many real situations in which several of the girls married a man similar to their father and several of the brothers did not want to be abusive but did ended up being abusive to their partner. This does dramatically demonstrate how modelling teaches so well?

I can give you many cases where the abused women had lost so much self-esteem that they were unable to get away from the abuse. I have actually been aware of some cases that ended up in tragedy with the murder of a wife in an abusive partnership. I also can give the rare example of the child that has 'made it' and has eventually; neither married an abusive partner or ended up being abusive themselves

I went on to elaborate another feature of "modelling". All of the things like how a parent must treat their partner, how to show affection, how to resolve problems, how to treat the children and so on; all these qualities are best shown by example.

A frustrated parent, often resorts to increasing the volume of their voices, in the misguided belief that it is a better way rather than discipline to get a message across, (it is often trying to avoid hitting the child). There are better ways to give the child a limit rather than hitting the child or yelling at them. Is the modelling that a frustrated parent should yell? So many parents ask me why yelling fails to work. I do explain that most children just learns to shut off listening to that parent; when it is their turn to be a parent they will use the same ineffective way (yelling) to try and discipline their children!

The genetics are so important that I have seen children that have been adopted of have been fostered turn out very similar to their biological parents. The early life experiences are also very important. The influence of peer pressure is not under the parents' control. The influence of good parenting means peers have less influence on the child's and the child does come back from those influences. I did say that good example means that that the child will choose peer that have a similar value system to their parents and so the peers go on influencing the young person in good ways.

I quoted what I discovered that children with ADHD do often turn to a drug habit but that they have a much better chance of kicking their habit and to go 'straight' if they have had a good childhood and their ADHD was treated properly than the people than those that had a traumatic childhood.

The meeting always ended, by the facilitator playing a tape of Chaplin's song "The Cat and the Cradle". That evergreen song completely summarized that children ended up like the example their father had given them.

CHAPTER TWENTY-FOUR

---◆》》·《◆---

The incidence of ADHD depends on which country figures you look at; it depends how they define the problem and how they look at it. Some countries define the problem as a psychosocial disorder; we define it as a biological disorder; I suggest that it may be neither; it may be a normal variant. No matter how it is described our children need help so they don't end up with bad self esteem.

The principals of management of all children are much the same; they are even more with children that have problems (such as ADHD Asperger's Syndrome and the many other psychological problems that children have. The child needs a lot of <u>loving, acceptance of the child, limit setting</u>, as well as being <u>protected, and being alerted to the dangers that lie ahead, prepare them for the future as best as we can and to help them reach their potential.</u> Always remember that we are have been entrusted with their care and that they are not our belongings. They are only on loan to us for several years.

I find an experiment by a man called Harlow very interesting; it is known as Harlow's monkeys. Monkeys are quite a social animal He compared the differences of behaviours adult monkeys that had different feeding experiences as infant monkeys from those that were brought up normally. He started to feed baby monkeys by a bottle held by a wire "mother": he found that those monkeys grew up as much less social than the normals. He then repeated the experiment with wire "mothers" that had a furry covering over the wire 'mother'. He found that those monkeys were better socially but still not as good as the monkeys in the wild. Next he fed some infant monkeys with the furry 'mothers" but he attached a tape recorder so that the "mother" made sounds like normal feeding mothers and made while feeding their babies. Those monkeys turned out as adults that were close to normal (socially).

This study demonstrated to me how important is mother's voice and touch is for the normal further development of an infant monkey. Mind you one has to be careful when we generalize animal studies.

Another study; that seems very relevant to this topic was done in South America; unfortunately that study was only done not using all the precautions of a 'double blind' medical study to ensure that bias does not occur. It demonstrated that a child- mother attachment did occur as soon as baby saw mother. That does raise questions what happens to sick babies when they don't see their mothers right away and they are immediately taken to the premature infant ward and probably placed into an insulcot. Any way most mothers have a very special bond with their children.

A further feature of animal behaviours which like human behaviour but not as inflexible is called imprinting, A duck is sitting on its eggs and the ducklings are about to hatch; just before the hatchlings make their way out of the eggs; the mother duck is taken away and dog is placed near the hatching eggs; the first thing the hatchlings see is the dog so they attach themselves to the dog. They follow the dog anywhere it goes'. Once it has taken force it cannot be change in ducks. In humans it is called a critical period. Most likely the child–mother attachment takes place then; but it is not so inflexible that once it has taken place it cannot be altered–again; it can but with a lot effort.

The simple principles of behaviour control are reward for wanted behaviour and the 'punishment' for the suppression of unwanted behaviours.

The principal of simple conditioning were first described by Pavlov. In his experiments; he trained his dogs to repeat their behaviour because of a primary reward–food; he would give his dog's food so they learnt to present at that time to get food; he later would ring a bell just before he would give the dogs food and his dogs started to salivate in preparation to eat. Very simply put; we reward the behaviour we desire from the child and we punish and so suppress the behaviours we don't want the child to produce.

The system that was preferred years ago was punishing bad behaviours. Remember that punishing unwanted behaviour will just result in the behaviour being suppressed. Hopefully the unwanted behaviour will eventually die with the passage of time Physical punishment if administered fairly and correctly has the advantage of being quickly and can follow quickly to the unwanted behaviour. If the child has bad memory problems it is very important that the child knows what the unwanted behaviour was and what the punishment was for.

If too much time elapses between the "punishment" and the behaviour being punished the whole point may be lost. In our country it is still acceptable to use physical punishment. It has to be below the waist, and not in a private area, the buttocks are a good place. It must not leave a mark, we should not use a weapon and it must not be given in anger. The danger of physical punishment is that it can be overdone as it is as often associated with parental frustration. I can think of times that (I was like the priest was supposed to have said "do as I say but don't do as I do". It was associated with a lot of anger and frustration. Children can be very forgiving provided it does not happen too often. There are so very many dangers to using physical punishment that some counties have banned all forms of physical punishment altogether, presumably that is because of the inherent dangers of physical punishment and it is a form of aggression. Mind you if we did have a machine that we could set to a level to deliver a painful stimulus to an appropriate level for the targeted misbehaviour it might be good, but this is not available. The reward system is now the preferred way to go.

Rewards can be primary rewards like sweets, or their favourite meal. They can be secondary like praise, their favourite outing, money or solo time with their parent.

Remember always that it is what the child wants; if it is to be a reward, not what we may consider that they want.

A points system can be set up; the child can earn point by fulfilling a task we want them to do. We allot the points according to the difficulty of the task or the difficulty that a child has to complete that task. The points that they earn are recorded daily and added up daily. When the child has earned enough points; the child can get the reward they chose; the rewards that were agreed upon. The progress is discussed with the child; if they are successful or why they are failing to achieve the wanted goal. Some of the reasons as to why the reward point system fails are; (a) Our expectation were set too high (b) Reading chosen for the child that hates reading because of a (perception) reading problem that they could not help. (c) The reward is not what they want but it is what we think they want. (d) It takes miles too long for the child to get their chosen reward. The timing does depend on the child's memory. The shorter the child's memory is the sooner the points have to be converted into the real rewards that they chose; it is useless for a child with a very short memory to wait for the term results to get their reward. There are many reasons why it can fail; I will discuss some more of these as I go on. As I said it is very important to ensure that a reward is actually what the child wants and not what we think should be a reward to the child. I often do come across the failure of a reward system that has been setup with a lot of effort. The child wanted money as their reward. They actually wanted what money could get them. However the parents' expected the child to bank what the child "earns". Commonly parents gave the answer that they wanted their child to get a saving habit. When I point out why their system failed is that the child did not appreciate a savings plan. Looking at a bank balance is not a reward to most children. For the parents that insist that the child saves what they "earn", I suggest that they bank half for the child or the child does it for themselves and the other half, they child gets to spend on whatever they want. Some children just choose to spend quality time with one of their parents, just on their own; without a sibling. It may be that they want to go shopping with their parent. Other children choose they would love to go to the beach, or to a family picnic or some other outing. The theme parks are often chosen as a wanted reward. The parent decide what behaviour that the child present with is the ones that they want to change they then draw up the chart rewarding the child for achieving a change of the unwanted behaviour to the wanted behaviours.

They must not choose too many behaviours at one time to try and change. It is preferable to choose two or three behaviour at one time To give you a real example that some parents chose; (a) keeping your room clean; (b) put your school away in the right place, and not just dropping it at the back door as you come into the door (c) do as your mother says the first time- not having to be asked repeatedly.

To expect an improvement of about one third reductions of the unwanted behaviours converting into wanted behaviours in 1 to 3 week is realistic but to expect a greater change is quite unrealistic. Watch out for an effect that I call "the honeymoon period". This is a change that can occur because the new system is novel not because it was chosen well. Another problem that can present is that the positive system works initially but then it fails to maintain the positive changes. The reason is usually that the child is testing the parents out to ensure that the changes in the management by the parents is real; will the parent fall back and return to the old system given some time. Are the changes really for real? In that case the therapist must encourage the parent (often they have been heavy handed) to persist with the positive rewards system. You can see there are many aspects to a change of management style to the reward system that you may need more input about.

The Positive Parenting system elaborates on the reward system and the reward chart, so for those parents that need more information about positive parenting they can be referred to the many Positive parenting courses that are available. Often schools and community services like the 'neighbourhood centres' offer these Positive Parenting courses.

Children are so intelligent and the danger is that they can use the fact that we don't want the behaviour so they can produce this defiant behaviour to annoy us. The young child with Opposition Defiant Behaviour is especially prone to defy us! Too many judgments are made using today's standards to judge the past happenings. Conditions were so different then. For just one example, there was no child support system so that girls that did not have parental support found it so difficult to keep their babies. Some babies were at risk of harm if they were not taken by children services. Was not adoption considered a good alternative at that time? The idea was to try and give a child a chance of a better life. The effect of separation from the mother was not jet understood. Making judgments using today's standard not if considering the real facts of the conditions in the past is seems so unfair if anything. I see so many dramatic reports that are made of thing that were suppose to have happened so many years ago, perhaps time have dulled the memory or wish fulfilment has altered the memories of what actually happened or why it has happened!

Do you recall that most of us grew up in much harsher times? For instance, if a child lost his shoes, often their parents could not afford to just get them another pair. These days, the parents will be upset, but they will get another pair and not let their child go without shoes. Just after the world war, times were much harder for most. Such things as rationing still existed in many countries. A lot of fathers returning from; the dreadful war; suffered with post-traumatic stress disorder. Many did not want talk their horrible experiences; to make matters worse; their problems were often not recognized. If they were recognized to be suffering with post traumatic disorder they were often ineffectively treated (if at all).

Years ago the condition was not recognized at all; some soldiers were shot because supposedly they did not have "intestinal fortitude"; later the army recognized that they suffering. The condition was first labelled "shell shocked" and today it is well recognized as post traumatic disorder.

I found recent research by the by the Vietnam returned soldier's section of the R.S.L to be very interesting. You can imagine how difficult it is to study brain of living beings, so most of the research depends on MRI's findings. They have demonstrated that there is an actual <u>anatomical</u> brain change in the brain of returned servicemen suffering with post-traumatic stress disorder. Many of their children have features of ADHD. The research is ongoing.

Again I repeat that Discipline or limits setting is extremely important for a child's normal development. It is even more important to a child with ADD or ADHD. Limit setting and predictability is the corner stone of a child's security. Experts in child psychiatry tell that consistency is essential and it is so important in a child's life. This is especially so, with young children. However as the children grow up consistency is not as important. It is important that children understand and experience of the variability in human reaction in different situations. That is humanity! It is not always predictable and consistent. The general way that we use the terms discipline it is for limit setting and every child needs limits. Whereas we use the term punishing to describe that it is for the benefit of the frustrated parent and not for the purpose of the child's limits setting. Take the example of a child that has just been punished; the child goes on and on crying (or demanding) in spite of the parent's request to stop; then the parent's frustration escalates. The parent reacts to the child's behaviour because of their frustration. They often resort to punishing the child again. Then they can overdo the discipline and then it does become punishment. The child may interpret that the parent's frustration is with them; that it means that the parent does not like them (not just their behaviour). Parents do try to counter that by telling the child 'I don't like your behaviour but I do love you. It may work, but it may not because feelings are stronger than words. The parent might apologies, but if this happens again and again in, the child may not really accept the apology. During times of frustration, the parent usually resorts to increasing the loudness of their voice in the hope that the parent yell may avoid the physical punishment. What is the modelling that is taking place? What does this modelling teach? Is yelling the way to go? This may effectively results in the child switching off and learning to take little notice or to do the same.

Let's me emphasis how important it is that parents pull together. It is so important that parents are aware of each other's advice and not to encourage the child to learn how to use one parent's advice against the other.

Parents should be very committed to each other; picture now that you are a traveller in the desert and you have not one but two guides. You ask the first guide 'what is the way that we should go' he tells you 'north, that way'. Then you check it out with the second guide and he tells you 'not to believe the other guide tells you; and to go west', so you decide not to trust either and go your own way! That is what it can be like for a child when the parents don't pull together; they give the child different advice (or they have different beliefs about discipline techniques) from each other. Parents that work hard to give the same advice or direction to their children find it so much easier to manage their children. They must show a good relationship. Each parent must demonstrate and show affection to each other, to the identified child and to their other children. Remember that a parent can't be a child's best friend and a guiding parent at the same time. This can be a real problem for some parents and can be especially difficult for single parents, trying to be mother and father at same time. I will now describe a very humorous incident, from my life. My very bright grandchild was five at that time; he is now a beautiful adult. He was having problems with eating his meals and he was underweight. His concerned parents discussed this problem and they decided that he would not be given anything to eat or drink for 1 hour before dinner, fair enough. Not long after their discussion, the boy asked his father for a drink of milk half an hour before dinner. Obviously, father told him"we told you, not before dinner". So he went to ask his mother who was busy preparing the meal. He kept on pestering her; as to how thirsty he was! She offered a small drink of water, but that would not do. He kept on pestering her still. So she finally gave in and said you can have ½ a small "vegemite" glass of milk. He drank it with relish! He then promptly went to his father and pointed his index finger at him and said "see I told you I would get a drink from mummy!" Naturally this prompted a reaction from father and a heated discussion followed with his mother! He still speaks out his mind and has a good value system, naturally as you can understand; I am quite biased. He still has a small appetite but he is quite healthy. Did his parents; as do so many parents; worry unnecessarily about his nutrition? Many ADHD and Asperger's children have "food fads" most children do get over them eventually. Unless they are very obsessional about their food fad" are and they have other obsession; one must not worry too much about them. On another occasion his parent were visiting us; at that time we were living in a low set house and the house windows faced a large verandah; I don't remember what the child did to deserve being chastised but I do remember the details that followed vividly. His father sent him into one of the bedroom; my wife told his father that room has a low window and the child will get out easily. His father replied "he won't dare"; but he did go to check on him after a short time. The child was not in the room and he had climbed out the window. His father was worried so he ran to his house very close by looking for this young child. My wife and I also went looking for him on our property. As we got to the car port we heard a giggle; we looked under the cars; he was pulling himself up from under one of the cars. When my wife told him to come out from under where he was he did. Then he laughed out loud I got him didn't I?

Limit setting cannot be compromised but do always apply these limits carefully, lovingly and effectively. Do not corner your selves with threats that you don't intend to follow or screams that are ineffective.

Genetic factors are very important but so is the role of upbringing.

Research with identical twins many years ago indicated that several features such as intelligence; physical looks and like and dislikes are genetic features whereas personality feature are more likely to be due to upbringing. My sons look exactly like me. They often think the same way as I do, they walk similarly to me. The girls in my family look a little like me and a lot like their mother. When my first son was about to be born my wife asked the obstetrician "is it a boy or girl: he replied "I can't see that part yet but he had better be a boy because if it is a girl it would be a very ugly girl he added his just like his father". Sometimes children that have been adopted or fostered are not brought up by their biological family (from a very early age) and yet you can see the similarities to their biological family when they do grow up.

Undoubtedly some behaviours are due to the upbringing including the modelling that they observed. For an example some children are just like their fathers committed to their partner or alternatively selfish or even abusive and controlling.

What did a girl experience during her upbringing? Did she like her mother? Did she like the way she was treated? What was the modelling of the behaviour she saw? Did she do further studies to better understand human behaviours. An example of these studies; these include the medical, nursing or the social science courses. Were they brought up with somebody else rather than their parent? I was involved with the foster parents association I often saw as the child grew up; early upbringing as well as the genetic factors expressing themselves in the child's behaviours;. I have been privy to boys that grew up just like their father, either good or bad. Girls that accepted abuse and thought that was normal because they had seen their mother treated in that way for years, they did not know any different. Some family that has several children; some are like the parent of the same gender, but can be so different. None the less some do have several of the features of their parents. So what is the balance between genetics and up bring? It would seem that very few can break the "cycle' of genetic factors or the critical periods of learning I will now talk of my habit which luckily is not genetic; the habit of pocking my tongue does not just happen now when I am concentrating; it first began that way but it is now my trade mark.

I am not as aware of poking out my tongue; as I do poke out my tongue without thinking. My wife has so many photographs were I have my tongue poking out. She has to make a special effort to make me aware if she does not want my photograph taken with my tongue poking out. As I am getting older and not thinking as hard, this habit is getting less of a problem but it still happens. I just happened to come out of the consultation room. When a lady pushing a pram came past my surgery; she stared at me, she then just pocked out her tongue, just like me! She was not quite sure of the name on the surgery door but did recall my habit; even though it was so many years ago; that I had seen her in the practice with the Department of Health the Division of Welfare and Guidance. She then came into the surgery and we then caught up on old times.

She did come to see me for medical consults to immunize her two young children while she was still in the caravan park. She got her brother, whom I had also seen years ago; he too came to see me. I have not seen either since she left the caravan park.

The use of threat should be avoided. The child learns that threat are useless; unless the parent follows through with the threat the parent can back themselves into a corner as it were; if they don't follow through the threat is toothless so to speak if the follow through the parent will often overdo the punishment as they become frustrated after many warnings Often my wife used to use the threat of a smack with a wooden spoon, thankfully she never had to use it; when she hit the kitchen table with her wooden spoon and the children knew that they had 'crossed the line' and their mother was very angry.

One Christmas my children offered to buy their mother some new wooden spoons as she has broken so many hitting the kitchen bench when she threaten them with the wooden spoon. My own school experience had many incidents of physical 'discipline' being used often. I was often late so my teacher would have me wait outside until the end of the first lesson. He would then call me and any of the many other children that had been even a few minutes late that had been waiting on the veranda. He would the proceeded to strap all of us that were late. He used a leather strap about one inch thick and some ten inches long. He would start by placing the strap behind his back and swinging from the strapping all the way, with a lot of energy, onto our outstretched palms. We then went to our seats. He would then walk up the aisle and knowing that the children that had been strapped would be sitting on their hand in attempt to quell the pain that they felt, he would reprimanded us and then ask why they were not working. He would then use a steel ruler, and hit the children on the back of the hands on their knuckles.

I did tell my parents' of this common occurrence of the strapping that I received; they said that discipline helped to make me a better man. Very many years ago, I do recall having had a conversation with my parents; about the time of when I was at school; that I was hit across the knuckles with the steel ruler after being strapped. My parents told me that discipline is what made me such a good person. I responded to my parents that perhaps I would have achieved more if I had had more confidence and not been suppressed so much by physical punishment. Could my parents have been wrong about the punishment that I revived at school been wrong? Could I have been wrong that the punishment made me what I am? Or was it my ADD that caused my poor self esteem; or was it made worse by those punishments? I have come across some dreadful cases of punishments that were actually child abuse; some children were punished with an ironing cord or a thick belt. In some other cases children were locked up in the boot of the family car over night. I was eventually mandated to report cases of child abuse; before that mandating I could face litigation because I broke confidentiality; luckily I never had to face litigations.

CHAPTER TWENTY-FIVE

━━━◀))·◀(((━━━

I will now discuss the many 'fads' have been proposed to treat the ADHD. I will start by discussing the FIENGOLD'S food sensitivity diet.

The ADHD child was supposed to be sensitive to naturally occurring salicylates. There are still many proponents of this diet. There are still volumes of many books that are published by and written by dieticians on this subject. Some dieticians have even got their doctorit (PHD) writing a thesis on the subject. In my opinion, this exclusion diet is useless. I was initially very impressed with the results that were claimed to result from this exclusion diet. I was very hopeful that it would work but I was terribly disappointed. At that time I was in charge of the Redcliffe clinic as the Medical Officer of the with the Queensland Health Department the Division of Child Guidance. The Division invited Professor FIENGOLD to visit the Divisions headquarters. He accepted the invitation to come to Queensland and talk to use about this diet. The Director of the Division asked all the Medical Officers in charge of the various clinics to prepare suitable cases to present to him. There were quite a few clinics of that Division at that time. As I said I was quite excited to present him cases of ADHD children in which his diet was successful. I was to be badly disappointed. I painstakingly explained the diet to the parents of properly diagnosed ADD and ADHD children. I made sure that the parents and the child did understand what food and drinks the child had was to be restricted from in their diet. The child could be challenged after being on the restriction diet for several weeks with a food or drink that contained salicylates; if the child was ok with that food then that food could reintroduce in their diet again. One item at a time could be reintroduced if the child did not become hyperactive with that food item. In that way the parent would find out what foods the child could and should not consume; so they would know what to avoid in their child's diet. After ten weeks on the diet I reviewed the results. Some children may have improved; perhaps it was that parents had impose some discipline- limits on their child or it could have been the novelty factor. However there were several children that the diet did not make any difference to their attention, distractibility and certainly no difference to their memory problem. Two children had actually decompensated with their behaviour; one had started to soil himself; while the other child started to wet his bed. Perhaps I had inadvertently given his parents' of the child that started to soil himself another "weapon" to control him further and that was why he started to soil himself. I had probably also inadvertently caused the child that started to wet his bed more anxiety with more restrictions.

Many of the other clinics had similar results to mine so again I say that I was so disappointed with our results. I got permission from the Division's Director to invite a Professor of nutrition from the University (QUT) to come to Professor FIENGOLD'S talks. The Professor that I had invited to the talk I did not really understand the technical answers that Professor FIENGOLD gave him and neither did I. The long and short of it is that the answers that the Professor that I had invited, got did not make sense to either of us. Our own NHMRC put out a statement, after reviewing the available research; that stated that after reviewing all the available data; they could not find any evidence that support or proved that diets made any difference to ADHD children. The main research article that the NHMRC depended on was an USA study. In this study the researchers took over the whole diet of a city of one hundred thousand people. Only the computer "knew" who was on the diet and which child could access what food (they did know that children often swap lunches). The observers did not know what child was on the diet, so observer bias was eliminated. After several weeks they compiled the results of their results. Remember that it was only the computer that knew who was on and who was not on the diet! The observers noted the children's behaviours; the observer reports about the child's behaviours could not know but their observation could reflect what child was on the diet and what child was not on a diet so they could not be considered biased. Furthermore it was only the computer that knew what children had broken their diets by swapping lunches, what children could have not broken their diets because they did not have access to foods that were not on their diets and so on. At the conclusion of the study the researcher put out a result that there was no evidence to support (or deny) that diet made any difference to ADHD.

It is undeniable that there are a few; but only a very few children; that are truly allergic to certain foods. I do not know if ADD children have a larger presentation because of allergy and that it is a larger percentage of the so called normal population. Many other things in a child's diet have been (falsely) accused of causing ADHD or at least avoiding these foods improved the child with ADHD's behaviour. Many colorings and preservatives have been accused of creating problems. Many drinks have been similarly accused of causing the child to be 'Hypo"; I think it should be "Hyper" as many parent say. Chickens are fed yellow feed to make their eggs more attractive to consumers. This yellow in the eggs was supposed to aggravate ADHD. The egg board called me to assure me that the yellow was made the from natural colour of maize and it did not contain salicylates

A similar belief is that sugar gives many people 'highs'. I find this contention very difficult to accept because we do have so many controls of our blood sugar levels; it is strictly controlled within certain levels. I know that I do feel like a snack or a meal when my sugar level falls below a certain level but I certainly don't become overactive; and the opposite is true. It is a disease when the controls fail and the sugar level does increase abnormally, it is called diabetes mellitus; but the patient is not hyperactive. There are other products that have come and gone and been initially 'fan fared' and claimed to treat ADHD. E.g. the A2 milk; some tea that I don't even remember what it was called; (fish oil-omega 3) that is still being researched and many chemicals like Pycnogenol which is the bark of some tree, have been claimed to treat or help in the treatment of the condition of ADHD. The condition of ADHD and so many other conditions are so common that many people see the dollar signs; so that desperate parents trying to help their children with those conditions children will try most things once. Once they have purchase their product, in the hope that the claims are correct; the makers of these products have your hard earned money and won't be giving it back. They laugh all the way to the bank with your money. There are many products that advertise on the internet that claim to treat or help in the treatment of ADHD or ADD and Asperger's syndrome. My advice is to save your money and don't try unproven remedies in the hope that they can help. Many dramatic reports fan the hope that these treatment are so wonderful and that they have proved effective. There are other claims that other things besides diet may help ADHD they are just as useless. You may recall that colored glasses were all in vogue one time? They were very dramatically reported on a television program. The colored glasses were supposed to help correct ADD reading problems. Some vulnerable parents; spent considerable amounts of time and money in the hope that this treatment would help their child. They too were disappointed. They were probably hoping that they could find an alternative treatment for their child's problem. I can understand how publicity and the word of mouth by the advertising machinery and the lobby of alternative treatments and the promise to the parents, desperate to help their children with learning problems can sell a solution to them. Often these problems are only a part of ADD or ADHD.

I will get back to the colored glasses. Ophthalmologists were the first to recognize and describe the visual learning problem that most ADHD children have. I don't believe that many fully understood the full complexity of the visual processing problems. They believed that some simple measure could correct the problem, colored glasses. When a report on went on air on a 'Current Affair'; many optometrists hopped on the band wagon and prescribed colored glasses. I do know of an ethical optometrist that loaned the parent prescription glasses to try to see if it did help the child before the parent bought the glasses. In our society, ADD or ADHD is such a common problem and the so called 'treatments' to correct the problem are numerous. I believe that because of the placebo effect the treatments seem to work; initially at least. Very few prove effective in the long run but only a few help the majority. Most of these treatments are quite expensive; money a lot can't afford but they do spend the money in the vain hope that it will help their child. Some treatment are cunning enough to say that the treatment will take some time to work so the child's parents buys more of the product hoping that eventually they see positive results alas. The concerned parents are easy prey and some continue to be so. Again I want to emphasis how complex the problem ADHD is be so a simple treatment that cures all manner of problems is bound to fail.

Another treatment that had its day was the repetitive exercise programs. Doman and Dellacatto, two American psychologists first described this as a treatment program for severely handicapped children. They called this system of exercise Patterning. This system involved giving the handicapped infant constant passive exercises, moving the child's body and limbs constantly. The child's parents often enlisted neighbours to be able to constantly "stimulate" the child; for hours at a time. It was such a fad that I do know of one desperate family trying to help their child mortgaged their house to go to USA and get an appointment with that institute. Incidentally the two psychologist spit when one partner discovered that the system they described did not work and the other partner was using it as a money making ploy. The fundamentals of this system were taken up by an exercise program for the ADHD children. A representative of this program came to my children's school to sell the exercise program to the school. It was a general exercise program for all the children. In my opinion, most of the children were now too old to benefit from this general program. I asked many searching questions at the evening meeting for the parents. As a result the school saved their money and did not buy the program. Exercise Physiotherapist and Occupational therapist do design individual exercise programs for <u>young</u> children that have coordination problems especially.

CHAPTER TWENTY-SIX

T he management of ADHD ADD and Aspergius depends on both giving the necessary advice for the problems that present and the appropriate medication if required. The treatment must not depend on medication alone; medication is an adjunct to the whole treatment. Most of the dramatic reports bagging the traditional medical treatment are the result of using medication alone and/or of poor follow up. The treatment depends, on the child's age at presentation and what symptoms you choose to treat. The advice I discussed in this book is necessarily of a general nature.

I emphatically give the advice that management has to start; for any child but even more so for child with any problem; for example ADHD. It is that it is of utmost importance that we must start by loving and accepting the child. This may be difficult at times, because of the child's difficult behaviour; which can be a result of their problem. Above all, always emphasis how you care and love them- remember their self-esteem. Families that have their own problems do complicate the child's problem; this is especially so when the mother has psychiatric problems that may include such things as unresolved post natal depression or just depression, schizophrenia or bi polar disorder. Often the fathers have their own problems and make the mother's problems worse. They may be aloof, non supportive or worse abusive. During the history taking we must have explored the family functioning. If there are problems in the families functioning areas they must be attended to. Relationship problems in the family are common; in this day and age and in our society. For instance; only about some 50% of marriages last today. Most families end up breaking up within two years of marriage. The families that have to deal with problem children are even more at risk of getting into trouble with their marriage because there can be to so many differences in parental opinion. There may be a multitude of difficulties in the family; like relationship problems, parental differences in how to manage the child's behaviour or parental disunity and inconsistencies with the "discipline". If it is possible I would try and refer the parents to a family therapist; however that is not always practical. So I have learnt how to be a family therapist myself. I do use an eclectic approach when dealing with family problems; I found that I'd often use the McMaster model of family functioning to deal with many problems of families as I find it very useful in so many cases. This model of family functioning was first described in 1984 however it is updated regularly. If you would like to find more about this model and the seven levels of family functioning; it is available on the internet. Just ask Dr. Google.

I will give another common example of problems that do occur; one parent may laugh at the child's defiant behaviour initially; but that parent may get very annoyed or even angry with the same behaviour as the child get older. Verbal disapproval is a common effective way to disapprove of young children behaviour. If that is not enough, a common technique is to use a naughty mat or chair; it is better to call the place you send the young child to by a better name rather than the naughty chair; potentially the child associates the chair that he is naughty- not his behaviour. Perhaps it could be called the thinking chair. The young child must never be sent away where they can't see their parent or they can become very upset. They must not be sent to their room; as their bedroom can become associated with punishment. With older children; the child can amuse themselves in their bedroom and so the idea of limit setting is lost. I repeat that some of these general management techniques that I have described are even more important with children that have added problems. It is important to <u>establish a routine</u> for any child but for ADHD children it is even more important. For example many children with ADHD Etc. may have the problem of <u>organizing</u> themselves or they may have terrible memory problems I did write about the obstacle course for very young children with <u>coordination and balance</u>. Many children have <u>physical problems</u> too; these include <u>anxiety, bowel, bladder and sleep problems.</u> Sleep problems are very common with kids that have ADHD. Medication and management of these problems is often necessary; in order to treat the whole problem not just the ADHD. I have discussed how some parent wants my treatment for their behaviour; however my treatment is directed to their basic problem which in turn is responsible for the child behaviours. I see the ADHD children present because of their symptoms and I want to treat those symptoms. These symptoms can include; some but often not all; <u>hyperactivity, tactile issues, sleep disorders, poor concentration</u>, the child can be <u>easily distracted, learning problems</u> which can be with <u>reading</u> or <u>maths</u> or <u>both, self care problems, problems, organizational problems;</u> to organize themselves; or such things as, <u>poor coordination</u> and or <u>balance, expression difficulties, temper control</u> and <u>emotional problems</u> which usually cause a <u>poor self esteem</u>. They may also have <u>self control, memory</u> and often <u>relationship difficulties</u> and <u>anxiety</u> (this is especially seen with

Aspergius syndrome). I have already stated that stimulant medication is rarely used in young children (for their hyperactivity).

I have stated that it is not uncommon for ADHD children to have the associated problems; like anxiety, bowel or bladder problems and sleep problems. Medications are used to the target these problems. I will now try to describe the management of a few of these problems.

(1) Hyperactivity.

This problem is a hallmark of ADHD. It is often associated with short concentration and high distractibility. The Child usually responds well to medication backed up with management. The medication of choice is Ritalin. I will discuss medication used for ADHD etc shortly. Routines, including meal times and sleep times are very necessary. Calling on the body's time clock is always useful. Try and engage the child in a quiet activity, especially before bed. Do not yell, but reason softly with the child to slow down. Do not be over concerned by their dietary habits they do not cause the child's hyperactivity.

(2) Poor concentration and Distractibility.

The symptoms of poor concentration and heightened distractibility often, but not always go together; with hyperactivity. Always ensure that you have the child's attention by getting eye contact, before talking to them or issuing a direction. It is better to do things with the child rather than expect the child to just do the tasks by themselves. For an example, it is better to help the child to stay on task by helping them to tidy their room; not than just to tell them to tidy their room; e.g. 'let's go tidy your room together before you go to your friends; they can and do get distracted by things that they may see and forget what they were originally doing if you are not there to keep them on task. As you can realize many symptoms are associated so the management of one problem often overlaps with that of another problem. Do not get annoyed with the child's problems at school, fighting, not remembering to bring some of their home work, because they were distracted by some other activity or child or they have ultra-short term memory problems too; so they just forgot to copy down the home work from the board. Often impulsivity is associated with distractibility so the child may hear from another child that another activity is so great that they 'forget' that the activity that they were so sure was the one that they wanted to do is not so great so they then want to change to the other activity. When the child wants to change their activity or join another club from the one that you spent so much money and time enrolling and setting them up for; at that time they were so sure that was what they wanted. Try to be firm and give them a full explanation of why it is so difficult to change now; point out that they may letting the old team down if they leave now; expect a lot of "buts: so keep your cool walk away if it gets to frustrating remember the teaching that you give your by modeling when you do back off. A good game to play with them, especially when in the car is the game of "I spy". It is a good idea to involve them in an active activity such as athletics or football. It not only helps with their activity but it may also help with their co-ordination and team work. Encourage them to join a Martial Arts Club, as this teaches self-control as well as self-defence. Support their ambition of an outside, manual or sporting occupation. Make the point that manual workers are needed by our society and the those occupations can be very highly paid.

(3). Learning problems.

As I have previously described <u>both visual and auditory</u> perceptual problems contribute to learning problems. There are many other names (labels) that are used to describe learning problems, for example; if a child's a reading problem that seems very severe, the parents can be told that the child has 'dyslexia'. Most often the problem is part of a bigger problem, so this diagnosis by name can further confuse the child's parents.

(a). <u>Reading problems</u>

This is such a large area that I will only intend to cover the main problems. I have described how if perceptual problems are present; they make it so difficult it is to recognize the symbols our alphabet. I have described how the many perceptual problems exist with the visual and auditory pathways. I have describes that one must start by making sure that both the visual and auditory acuity are normal, if there are any concerns for the health of the eyes at the original examination an ophthalmologist consultation should be arranged. Similarly the hearing has to be good. When one of my son's behaviours would go right off; my wife would suspect that there was a problem with his ears; he would not complain of sore ears. She would stand behind him and call out allowed "do you want a lollie. If he did not respond; she knew that his hearing was bad. It would mean that she had to take him to consult with the ENT Surgeon. He did end up needing grommets placed in his ear drums to drain the pus. When she picked him up from the hospital he told her "I can hear the birds singing".

Repetitive learning is the main way that perceptual problems that are corrected. Flash cards are often suggested one starts with simple words three or four letters than we precede to more complicated words as the child gets it correctly, (the majority of times). I always recommend, if it is possible, that the learning process is associated with fun activities. A reward system should be established for the child attempting and the compliance with the learning program every night. Be very careful not just to use this system to succeed with their reading. Remember that the child can't help their reading problem so you can encourage the child to try to read and not to avoid reading but don't get annoyed by their repeated mistakes or them trying to avoid reading; if you had a problem with reading you too want to avoid reading and not getting things right. The parent should read to the child as the child looks on. It is important to try and read to children every night and probably the same passage. Because many children have reading problem as well as memory problems; for them it is very important to repeat the passage that we read to them. Repetition is probably the only way I know to deal with learning problems; the hope is that eventually they learn the words by sight Obviously the child with both perceptual and memory problems has double the difficulty. I again always recommend that it reading time must be a fun time! Be sure that it is fun to your child; as what is fun to one child may not be fun to another. There was a fashion that schools used that was called "spellathons". Schools used to use these spellathons to raise funds. At one time we did sponsored several children for their spellathons; before we realized how terrible they were for children that had learning disability. When the children came to collect the money; you should have seen the poor child's face that had only got very few words right. My wife and I were not very popular when we raised this topic with the parent's and friends committee. We objected very adamantly to this practice by schools of raising funds; we told them it was belittling to the children with learning problems; anyway it was the parent's responsibility to raise funds not the children's responsibility to raise funds. They saw our point and that school no longer has spellathons. A simple technique that is helpful with the child that keeps loosing the place that they were reading from is to place a ruler below the line they are reading so that the line below is covered With children that get confused with the spaces between words and the words seem to run into each other; a simple card cutout which only allows one word at a time to be demonstrated can be used. (One word at a time only is displayed). Many children do eventually mature past these problems; however if we don't help the child in the mean time; damage can and will result while we wait.

Many children are quite compliant; but it does depend on the personality of the child; if they are we can use that quality to draw upon. E.g. a careful competition with a sibling with similar competence is used for used to encourage them to learn. Great care has to be used when using this as a method to encourage the child as the sibling can taunt the patient with their poorer results. There are now several services that assess the perceptual problems but I am not aware that they provide a program to correct the problem that they identify. There are some experimental programs that are trying to correct the problem. I do emphasis that they are experimental and not yet proved and they are often quite expensive. There have many organizations that offered treatments for these problems but they all are quite expensive and non effective; many have come and gone as parents have found that the promise the organizations made were not delivered. In any case these organizations have got and banked your money and it is now in their account. I do sound very biased but I don't make any excuses for my dissolution.

(b) <u>Mathematics</u>.

The same perceptual problems exist with the numerical symbols of mathematics as there are with the alphabetical symbols. The same principles are effective to correct these problems. One of my children did have such a problem; He overcame his difficulty with the repetitive leaning of "Kumon Maths". I am good at maths so the night before his grade 10 final examinations he asked me to help him. I had not helped him before as it is commonly said 'the plumber family's leaking taps are the last thing that gets fixed by the plumber'. Just as well, I had not helped him before, because I found myself getting very frustrated as I tried to explain simple mathematic principles to him. He had learnt maths by simple rote learning and not by basic understanding. I quickly realized that trying my way would only result in more frustration and eventually yelling. So I decided to desist and try to 'break the ice' and ask him to answer a riddles. The riddle goes like this. 'If an electric train is travelling north at 30 mph and the wind is blowing south at 20 mph, in what direction and at what speed would the smoke be travelling?' He immediately got it. He said "Dad there would not be any smoke if it was an electric train!" I continued with the mathematics tutorial using only examples that appealed to him. He achieved a satisfactory pass in his grade ten examination.

(4) Tactile.

While I was a resident at the Geelong Hospital; on the occasion that Evelyn has to have an operation I was working as the acting paediatrician on call; my infant child was only several weeks old so he was admitted to the children's ward. When the charge sister was having trouble feeding my infant child they called the paediatrician on call which happened to be me! The ward sister was disgusted with me because I wrapped the child up; put him down in his cot on his side and put the bottle in his mouth. He started feeding happily. I did explain to her that he hated being touched so it was no use trying to cuddle him. He still does not like very close cuddles for a long time. I will talk later of some very interesting research that was well done. How relevant are these research articles to our children with ADHD etc? These articles are about Harlow monkeys and the duck's imprinting and our critical periods? What are the consequences for the child that has ADHD?

(5). Self–care.

This can be a common presentation. It is often due to a memory problem, the child simply forgets to look after themselves. A very funny presentation was of a parent complaining that the child's underpants always had skidies in spite of the parent's directions. It turned out that the child was often in a hurry so he forgot to wipe his bottom properly (or to wash his hands). When the child grows up they become interested in the opposite gender so usually they start to be very interested in there self-care.

(6).Expression difficulties.

I am personally familiar with this problem as I have had that problem all my life. In secondary school my teachers would say to me "I think I know what you mean but I am sure that people that don't have any idea of what you mean". I have had to expand my descriptions in this book several times, so that you do understand what I mean. I have learnt; over a long time; that my problem was the précis of my ideas, so much so that the missing parts resulted in the idea not making any sense. I am often ahead of myself so I put the later thought first and then the second thought Good teachers are invaluable' they know their pupils understand them and can then point out what their problems are and then how to correct them.

(7).Co-ordination.

This problem results in clumsiness, balance problems and poor sporting abilities.The exercise programs, a referral to a physiotherapist, joining sport club, joining Martial art club, encouraging physical activities and joining a sports club all help to improve the co-ordination. However some problems persist and as a result some individuals are not very interested in sporting activities I have describe the early interventions with the obstacle course that I used!

(8) Memory.

Memory actually has 4 different aspects to it. It has ultra- short term, short term, intermediate term and long term memory. Then we also have another skill called-recall (of stored memory). Ultra-short term memory is an electrical property. It depends on the axon having a branch dendrite which returned to the initial axon thereby resulting in a reverberating circuit. The dendrite stimulates the axon keeping the axon active. An example of this memory function is recalling what is written on the blackboard long enough to write it into our exercise book. You can realize the difficulties that a child faces when they have an ultra short term memory problem

Short term memory results when a connection between axon and adjoining dendrites takes place; it does so by a weak protein bond between nerves. An example of this is remembering what you had for breakfast today. In Korsekoffs psychosis (because of heavy alcohol intake) patients lose their short term memory. They make up stories for their missing memory and what's more they believe their stories.

Intermediate memory is established when a RNA bond between the neurons is laid down; an example of this memory is remembering things that occurred several day or weeks ago. For example what you did on your recent holiday. Long term memory is a firm DNA bond between neurons. An example of this is do you remember your "honey moon" if it was some 50 + years ago? With dementia; patients they start being aware of the difficulty in recall and memory, and then as a result they get anxious. However they then forget what it is that they forgot so that they don't worry. The pattern goes on; they then lose more and more memories. They start loosing their short term memory then there intermediate memory. There long (very long term memory) is the last to go. They remember things that happened to them many years ago, eventually they forget even their children's names and even later they don't recognize them. We still don't know all there is about dementia but we do know that in some cases there is a genetic basis for the condition.

Returning now to the child with ADD and ADHD; they often have ultra-short term memory and short term memory problems. You can understand the difficulties the child faces at school; school depends on learning and memory. What is the difficulty that a child faces if he or she can't remember what is on the black board long enough to copy on their book? What happens to their self- esteem and motivation to study all evening if by the next morning they have forgotten everything that they learned the night before?

A simple game is available called simple memory; it consists of a set of cards; two cards have a picture of the same thing e, g. an animal. The cards are first shuffled then they are placed face down. The child picks two cards to match them if they do they get to keep the cards if they don't match the cards are returned face down. The child has to recall the cards location in order to match them. The game is usually made more interesting by competing with a parent or another child. The game can be more complicates by the same animal is presented but now it can be in a different colour or position but another pair is correct. The person that gets the most pairs wins the game.

Again the game of "I spy" is a good way of encouraging remembering objects that we see or we can recall from memory and we can see them; it is associate to the letter that the object or action starts with; so not only you have to guess what object the other person is thinking about but you have to work out from the clue; what letter that object start with

(9) Temper.

Many children with ADD or ADHD or Aspergius have a quick temper. Children with Aspergius often suffer with great anxiety, so if they are put into a position that does not seem; to them; to have an alternative response, they often react with anger. E.g. Scream, hit the teacher or child that upset them; they can even resort to throwing a desk across the class room. They can react very impulsively

It is often said of ADHD children are like: as a common bumper bar sticker reads "put your brain into gear before they open their mouth".

ADHD children often cannot stay out of things and they can be very impulsive so they can be easily 'set up'. It is stated that other children know that ADHD children react quickly so they can make the bullets and the ADHD child fires them.

(10).Emotional.

Most children with any problem have emotional problems. ADHD and Aspergius children often have poor relational skills; although some are very popular. They seem to gravitate to children with similar problem, probably because those children are the ones that can accept them because they have a similar problem and they do understand each other? They are often caught misbehaving, they readily admit to the misbehaviour but they rarely explain the reasons as to why. Sometimes it can lead to double punishment for the same incident, first the school then the parent. They are so often in trouble, add to that their learning problem that results in poor school results, probably a memory problem and perhaps their poor relating difficulty. Make it even worse they are compared to a sibling or friend with good results. Is it any wonder that they have a poor self-esteem? They can be tortured with that poor self-esteem all of their lives even after they have learnt to adjust to their problem. It is very important to minimize the damage to their self- esteem; if their damage to their self esteem is to be minimized, the parents must shower them with **unconditional** love. Then the school teachers must like or better, love the child, and eventually that their employer must be understanding and be patient and praise their good work as well as show them how to correct any mistakes (repeatedly often). Their parents as well as their teachers must reward the child for trying and not just succeeding.

CHAPTER TWENTY-SEVEN

I will describe the medications that are commonly used to treat the various symptoms that ADHD and Asperger's children present with. Remember that the parent often wants that the child's behaviour is changed but we the practitioner aim our treatment and management to the symptoms and signs of the condition.

(1) **Methylphenidate** (Ritalin, Attena)

NMHRC put out a paper that Ritalin is the drug of choice to treat the hyperactivity, distractibility and concentration difficulty that ADHD have. The medication is a stimulant, so why use a stimulant with an already hyped out child? I will refer you to a very interesting research that was done at the start of the last century. Briefly the research studied 100 children that were diagnosed, not by one but by two child specialists; they were then compared to a control group of 100 children that were not considered to have ADHD. A PET scan was used to show the anatomical areas of the brain; and at the same time it demonstrated the areas that were active. This study made the assumption that the more active parts of the brain had a bigger blood flow at the time and so the color was red whereas the areas that had less blood flow at that time where blue. I considered this a reasonable assumption. The children that had been diagnosed with ADHD first activated the action parts of their cortex and a fraction of time later activated the frontal areas of the brain. The frontal areas of the cortex are the control areas. So what the bumper sticker reads is perfectly true of what ADHD children do. They act before they think of the consequences of their actions. It explains well why stimulation that act especially to activate the frontal lobes; the control cortex is put into action by the stimulants; so that is why stimulants work. Stimulating the control parts of the brain so that they are acting before the action takes place. So the ADHD child can think before they act when they are on a stimulant. Ritalin works for some 4 hours only. There are now long acting forms of Ritalin available on the NHS for school children only. Adult still suffering with ADHD cannot access this preparation even though they may be studding. They can however access the normal preparation. The main common side effects of Ritalin are the growth retardation and the appetite suppression. Very rarely there can be catastrophic blood pressure increases. Monitoring the child or adult that is on Ritalin requires that the blood pressure, growth and height are measured at every regular review. There are a few nuisance side effects with all drugs and especially stimulant e.g. headaches and nausea.

(2) Dexamphetamine

This medication was only one that was available on Australian NHS before Ritalin became available on our NHS. I still have some patients that were satisfactorily treated for their ADHD with this stimulant medication and I have not changed them over. The old saying that "when on a good thing stick to it" applies. In fact, some patients responded better to dexamphetamine than they did to Ritalin. Of course vice versa is also true. It has the same side effect profile as that for Ritalin. Perhaps it has more appetite suppression in some patients; if is taken to close to sleeping often results in being unable to go to sleep. Amphetamine, or speed as it is called on the streets; is used by many truck drivers as a preparation to stay awake. A derivative of speed is still marketed as an appetite suppressant and as a weight loss medication. I was very nervous of starting children on speed; was I starting a child on an addictive substance? At a conference on another medication; I spoke to visiting American child psychiatrist of my concerns, he told me not to be concerned and he referred me to then several paper that reported on several recent researches. The long and the short of those research articles was that children with ADHD are more likely to use illegal drugs but if they if they had been treated properly; they (would not have faced rejection and poor self-esteem and so not be anti authority); they are more likely to be able to kick their drug habit and return to a normal life. They may be even able to avoid drugs all together; whereas an improperly treated child with ADHD is more likely to continue with their drug habit and they are less likely to be able to kick their habit.

If the appetite suppression is a problem or the child stopped growing a common practice is to discontinue the stimulant medication at weekends. However, if it is possible; it is better to continue the medication even at weekend. There are so many social things to learn at weekends (as well as the academic things that they learn at school.

(3) Strettera. (Atomexatinde)

This is a non-stimulant, stimulant preparation; it is being used by many specialists; I have not used it much and therefore I don't have that much experience using it. It is not supposed to have as many side effects as the traditional medications have but I do like to wait until a drug has been out for a while before I make any judgments on the drug; then again I have not seen many side effects from the more traditional treatments. My early opinion is that it is slow to get the wanted results; and I personally did not continue prescribing when patient came back to me from specialists.

(4) Aurorix (moclemide)

It is a Rima (reversible inhibitor of monoamine oxidase) anti-depressant. This medication can be useful when the treatment using the traditional treatments for the hyperactivity expressed by ADHD children have failed. A study in Melbourne, of children, that were diagnosed with ADHD whose traditional treatment had failed to control their hyperactivity, poor concentration and their distractibility. Unfortunately, it only studied 25 children. It was quite effective in over 60% of those children where the traditional treatments had failed. It also showed some (minor) improvement in another 20% the children studied. I have also used it with patients that failed to respond to the traditional treatments and I had a partially successful result. There are some precautions with this medication as there are some potential interactions with other anti-depressants. This medication is also sometimes useful for other conditions including depression and weight loss.

(5) Catapress (clonidine)

It is primarily a blood pressure medication; the usual dose of the tablet is 150 milligrams. It has been also been found to be a useful treatment for migraine headaches. The tablet that is used for ADHD is only 100 milligrams and it is a very small tablet. I have empirically found that Catapress helps the heavy anxiety that most Asperger's syndrome sufferer have. I do have to start this medication very slowly as it can cause a large drop of blood pressure; it is a very small tablet; I do start with a quarter of a tablet for the first week then increasing by a quarter of a tablet every week it can be quite a pain because it is such a small tablet but slowly titrating is essential. It does make sense that a blood pressure medication that cause the dilatations of the blood vessels results in the improvement of the circulation of the frontal control center and as a result helps ADHD children to think before they act. Many paediatricians used this medication before the stimulants were approved as the first line treatment. I rarely; find this medication useful on its own; however I do find it very useful in combination with other medications; I often use it to support stimulant medications. I often use it for sleep problems that are very common in ADHD. A research that was first done by French scientists was very relevant in sleep problems (especially that ADHD children have). They did the research study, using healthy university students. They were allowed to sleep as long as they liked; however they were hooked up to an EEG (electroencephalogram) that was in turn relayed to a machine that would ring a loud bell as soon as they went into REM sleep.

Naturally the students were keen to join the study and get paid to sleep. Our human sleep consists of 4 phases. They are light sleep, then we fall into deep sleep, then we enter REM sleep then we go back into light sleep; we then repeat the cycle, in about 90 minutes. It is called REM sleep because during this phase of the sleep cycle we go through several bodily functions like our eyes moving from side to side hence the name Rapid Eye Movements or REM. Once awake we cannot go straight back into REM sleep; we can try to shorten the deep sleep cycle before we go into REM sleep phase but we cannot go into REM sleep straight away. We don't recall anything unless we wake during the REM phase. Occasionally we do wake during the REM phase and then we remember our dream however we do rarely go back to the same dream.

Dreaming does not really have the dream interpretations that are commonly attributed to dreaming. Dreaming either results from getting a somatic stimulus such as we need to go to the toilet, or reviewing the day's feelings and experiences. It was very interesting that these healthy students, both psychologically and physically did become very psychologically disturbed when deprived of REM sleep. After a period of REM sleep deprivation they became quite psychotic. When they were allowed to return to normal sleep they recovered fully. This does clearly demonstrate how important healthy sleep is to behaviour. We are now learning how important sleep-deprivation is. Several occupations suffer with sleep deprivation; doctors are responsible for people's lives. Sleep deprivation studies are also highlighting the issues of that nursing mothers face because they are deprived of normal sleep. Sleep apnea is now recognized and has to be mandatory reported if truck driver suffer from it. Some research indicates that it is a cause of depression.

Many children with ADHD and Aspergius have sleep problems. What does sleep deprivation cause to ADHD children's behaviours? I usually prescribe the stimulant medication earlier in the day so by the time night time arrives the stimulant has been metabolized Remember that both Ritalin and Dexamphetamine are short acting (4 hrs) even the long acting preparation for school kid only acts for 6 hours. Very occasionally I have had to prescribe stimulants for an ADHD child just before bed so that they get control of their hyperactivity and are then able to sleep.

Most of my friends find that if they drink coffee soon before bed they find it very difficult to go to sleep; but I find that a coffee just before bed gives me a good night's sleep. Coffee is a mild stimulant is that further proof that I have residual ADHD?

(6) Sertraline (Zoloft)

This medication is a major anti-depressant it is from the group of anti depressant called SSRI's. It is supposed to increase the serotonin levels in the brain; low levels of the chemical known as <u>serotonin</u> are responsible for depression. It is approved for major depression and for children that suffer from <u>obsessive compulsive disorders</u>. It is also very useful for the anxiety and the associated major depression that ADHD and Aspergius syndrome children suffer. Most children with ADHD or Asperger's syndrome are very much at risk of developing major depression It does have the typical side effects of the SSRI's. These are all listed in the product information that inserted by law in every pack. Care must be taken when prescribing this medication; as it does for all medication; to enquire what else the child is taking. For instance St John's Wart is like another weak is SSRI. Adding another SSRI to already taking an SSRI can result in Serotonin syndrome, luckily I have never seen it.

(7) Fluvoxamine Fluoxetine etc. (The other SSRIs, such as Luvox and Prozac)

I have already described one of the medications in this group. These are the new anti-depressants, namely the SSRI. They are very good as major anti-depressants and are very good to deal with anxiety.

Many ADHD and Aspergius sufferers suffer with major depression. Children can and do suffer with major depression. I wonder how many 'accidents' are actually child suicides? I did write about the child that was found hung on a clothes line; was at really an accident? Many children with ADHD and other problems in our society go on to suffer bipolar disorder, obsessive actions and thoughts, alcohol and drug induced psychosis. This is especially likely if they use "ice "methamphetamine. The manufactures of these medications warm about the risk of increasing depression and the risk of suicide especially with adolescents. Thankfully I have not seen anybody with suicidal thoughts or attempting suicide and with increasing depression. There is also a warning that people taking these medications should not drink however I see many that do drink (alcohol). They report that they need less alcohol to get inebriated. Many patients on these medications have an increase of their prolactin level. I have come across a patient that started lactating, however, as most patients do not suffer with any symptoms as a result of the increase prolactin level in their blood tests. There are many other antidepressant some are called SNRIS short for serotonin noradrenalin reuptake inhibitors of serotonin. Apparently our brain makes serotonin; but as time goes on we become more efficient so we don't waste anything and so we reabsorb the serotonin before it has a chance to do its work ; the SSR's inhibit the serotonins reabsorbing and thereby allows it to work before it is reabsorbed. It is of interest that many adult psychiatric wards were on the first floor; the hospital administration had to move the wards to the ground floor because they found that as soon as they stated to treat the badly depressed patients and they started to get better; they would jump out the first floor window. Apparently they were initially too depressed to do anything about how bad they felt but as soon as they started to feel a bit better because of effective treatment they did do something about how terrible still they felt and jumped out the window.

(8) Benzodiazepines; Valium (diazepam), Xanax (aloprozalolam) and the many Australian generics like Antenex, and the like.

These medications are very effective to treat anxiety in the short term.

Unfortunately they soon become very addictive in the longer term. The dose needed to reduce anxiety symptoms quickly escalates as tolerance and addiction take place. They are addictive and the sedation effect increases if alcohol is used with them. Some patients find that the medication is very useful and continue to use the medication at the recommended dose and don't become addicted.

They can be continued on this medication with close observation if tolerance and dose escalation is not a problem. Children's medication is nearly always controlled by the parents so over use is generally not a problem however it may stop working for some. I do often tell the story how a small pharmaceutical company first formulated this preparation; (Valium) as a result of making this very effective anxiolytic; the company became one of the largest pharmaceutical companies in the world. A first was this drug was claimed to be the wonder drug and many copies were made; later that the additive qualities and how addictive this medication can be. Is it because it allows for the anxiety symptoms to be controlled and the original cause of the anxiety is not addressed? There are now many copies (generics) of the medication available. I want to make a special mention of **Xanax** (The Australian brand is Kalma) it has the same problem of addiction of all the other drugs in the same group so it has to be closely monitored however it is the medication of choice when the other anxiolytic fail to control panic attacks. These medications are used for adults and they are only rarely used for children.

(9) **Sulthamine** (Ospolot)

This medication was used by the bucket load in years gone by; it is a German drug that promised to help ADHD; when the condition was called Minimal Brain Dysfunction; however the drug wholesalers are unable to import it any longer It was effective for some and it is supposed to especially help with memory problems. The results were quite satisfactory for some; but they were disappointing for others. I did see a child with ADHD and he also had a large increase of salivation, I don't know why but his salivation was totally controlled with Ospolot. When I tried to deal with his salivation without Ospolot his salivation was worse so I had to start it again.

Sometimes I have been totally frustrated because all traditional treatments failed. I tried Ospolot both on its own and with traditional therapy and it worked so I continued the medication. My local chemists accessed this preparation for me as some wholesalers still had some supplies of the medication even though they can no longer import it. I never did encountered any annoying side effects.

(10) **Carbemazine** (Tegretol)

It is an anticonvulsant. It is especially useful for focal epileptic conditions such as Temporal lobe epilepsy. It is very effective as a mood stabilizer for bipolar depression for some. This medication can be very useful for two symptoms especially, anger and occasionally with improvement of memory. It may help children with ADHD with their sea sawing moods. Unfortunately it does interact with many other medications so it has to be used with great care and with close observations for any side effects or interaction. It is often very sedating.

(11) Sodium valproate (Epillun and the Australian generic, Valpro)

They are often used to control epileptic convulsions. I do use these medications for ADHD occasionally. I do use them also as a help for the labile moods that some children have. In the cases of epilepsy the blood levels are important but in my cases of ADHD that I do use it with; a a low dose is usually adequate. The blood levels do not seem so important; as they are for epilepsy control. The dose that works effectively is usually is adequate enough. It is supposed to help memory problem however I have not found a medication that works for everybody and every time. I have found it very useful for epileptic conditions but I don't often use it because of its potentially bad side effects especially if the dose builds up into a toxic level.

(12) Amitriptyline (Tryptanol or the Australian generic like Endep)

There are many Tricyclics like Tofranil, Nortryptaline and Tetracyclic that are especially used for of the anxiety depression of Aspergius suffers.

Bed wetting can be quite a problem for the children that bed wet; they find it so embarrassing that many avoid "sleep overs" or school camps.

I still do use Tofranil for enuresis (bed wetting) as it produces immediate results. It allows the child to go to school camps or their friend to stay overnight. I am not sure how it works. It may be just a placebo that allows the child to be confident that they have treatment for their enuresis, on the other hand it may be a central effect; the control area in the brain that controls the bladder emptying when the bladder stretch reaches a certain point; or it may prevent the bladder emptying by resetting the urinary bladder's stretch reflex that causes the urinary bladder to empty; It may be a local effect that it allows the urinary bladder to stretch more, before an automatic reflex causes it to empty. The main problem with the tricyclic is that they can prolong (lengthen) QT segment of the heart's rhythm this is best seen on a cardiograph tracing; simply the drug can cause severe heart arrhythmias. It is essential that the child's heart is thoroughly examined, that usually involves a cardiograph; followed by a cardiologist consultation if any doubt still exists.

The urinary bed alarm has taken over the old thinking that enuresis was an emotional problem. The bed wetting alarm consists of a mat that is placed under the child sheets on the child's bed. The mat is actually two layer of foil so that as soon as the child starts wetting the urine completes an electrical circuit; which is relayed to a loud alarm. The loud alarm only goes off when the child starts wetting the bed thus completing the circuit. It is supposed to associate wakening the child to an unwelcome stimulus. Eventually the child learns to control the urinary bladder. The theory is that the alarm wakes the child but some children sleep so deeply that they sleep through the alarm; while the whole household is wakes up. The alarm should result in the child stops wetting the bed in about 12 weeks. I do want to again mention the dangers of the common practice of using a reward system for the successful achievement of a child stooping bed wetting (enuresis). If the child can't help wetting the bed they even feel worse if they fail to achieve their reward as well as feeling bad about their enuresis. They cannot help there enuresis until they are ready to do so. We don't start to even treat enuresis until the child is at least 7 years old;

There is probably a genetic factor to when we are ready to control our bladder

I will now discuss more of the treatment of enuresis.

(12) Desmopressin acetate. (Minirin nasal spray and it is now available in tablets form). Enuresis is quite common in all young children. As I said we do not start to treat child for enuresis until they are about seven years old.

Earlier the problem was considered immaturity and the treatment of choice was a tricyclic like Tofranil. It was believed that they relaxed the bladder and blocked the automatic reflex that emptied the urinary bladder when it stretched to a certain level. Apparently it allowed the cortical part of the brain to take control. This theory is no longer believed. The theory is now that child's kidneys make more urine at night. So the first line of approach to treating enuresis is the training of the child to hold on longer by way of the bed alarm. If the bed alarm fails then the next treatment is Minirin. It is a hormone treatment that directs the kidneys not to make urine during the night (while Minirin it is being used). During the day the Minirin has been metabolized so the kidney starts to catch up and get rid of collected fluid and so makes the urine. I personally don't like the idea of blocking the kidneys dealing with retained fluids. I do think that there is still a place for the past treatment (with the necessary precautions) with Tricyclics. While I am on this topic of bed wetting I should talk about the terrible habit of the common practice of (a) getting the child to take their night clothes and sheets to the Laundry or worse to wash's them too. (b) Punish the child for wetting the bed, in no way can the child help it. (c) To make a fuss and reward the child for dry nights; does show the child how much we want a dry bed and if they fail have they have let us down?

(d)I have already spoken of the dangers of a well meaning but flawed idea of a reward system.

If it does work well it is not our system that works but it is because the child is ready to do so

(13)Olanzapine, Risperadal (Zyprexia, Rispidol)

These medications are called the atypical antipsychotics because they less likely to cause side effects than the ordinary anti psychotics. The main side effects that are seen are a Parkinson like syndrome of stiffness and/or tremor; these symptoms are easily treated and fully reversible; either by stopping the medication or by using another medication.

The most concerning non reversible problem with antipsychotics is called Tardive dyskinesia. It usually starts with a fine quiver of the tongue. This drug is only approved by the NPS (subsidized prescriptions) for certain conditions in Australia. They include schizophrenia and the initial stabilization of bipolar hypomania. So its use for ADHD is quite expensive. I did consult a specialist in WA that does use it effectively for ADHD. Most Asperger's sufferers do benefit from this medication (if they can afford it). My experience with this medication is limited because most parents can't afford the price of the medication if is not subsidized.

(14) Several other medications that are used for these children. They are not for used for these children exclusively; they do also affect other children.

A**. Cyproheptazine** (Periactin). It is an antihistamine; in Australia it is approved for subsidized prescriptions for migraines prevention. It is reasonably cheap and it is a good appetite stimulant and it is effective anti-histamine. Other anti-histamines are commonly used for many children with ADD as many suffer do with many allergies; Nasal allergy and as nasopharyngeal rhinitis partly responds to antihistamines. Anti-histamines are quite effective especially with younger children as a sleeping medicine. However there is now a warning with antihistamines that they should not be used for children before they are 2 years old and for some antihistamine not until they are 6yeas of age. They can cause respiratory depression in some children.

Phenergan is a sedating antihistamine that is often used as a sleeping medication for young children.

(b) **Vallergan** (trimerprazine also know as in some counties alimemazine)

Is an appetite stimulant for some but it can also suppress appetite in others. Some children could be so underweight that weight gain is the main reason for their treatment.

(c)**Bisacodyl** (Ducolax Bisolax Parachock.)

Constipation is especially prevalent with Asperger's and some ADHD children. I often refer the serious cases to specialists for their bowel problem.

The Bowel Specialist check to make sure that their bowel problem is not of a more serious bowel problem; if it is not they are in turn often refer the child onto an occupational therapist.

Occasionally they require the aid of a rectal enema. If you would like to know more details about these medications, the internet provides the prescribing information (PI) for all of these medications.

Chapter Twenty-Eight

⟶»·«⟵

I will briefly summarize what I covered in this book. I started with a biography; after talking to some people that expressed that they were interested in people's experiences. I decided to combine my passion with some of my life's experiences so that I would reach a bigger base for my book. I was born in Egypt; I started by sharing some of my meager experiences of my early life. I then proceeded to describe my coming to Australia. Then I talked of my school years and then my university course. I completed medical degree at Melbourne University. I did my clinical years of my medical course base at ST Vincent" Hospital. During those under graduate years I was required to attend the other training hospital; namely The Royal Melbourne Women's hospital and the Royal Children's Hospital. During the under gradate years I met my wife. I did my residency at Geelong hospital where they prepared me well for my next venture in New Guinea. I was there for two wonderful years and I shared with you some of the different experiences. On my return to Australia I returned to Melbourne before I started with the Health Department of Queensland: the Division of Child Guidance. Before I started there; the place that I was to start at burned down so I did a locum for several weeks until the Department found me a place to work from. It was there that my interest in ADHD and child psychiatry flourished.

That Department is now Child and Youth Mental Health Service-CYMHS for short. After initially being trained for the position

I remained with that Department for many years and ended up in charge of the Redcliffe clinic of that Department. Financial and the family's needs; as the family grew; resulted in my leaving the Department progressively. I started in a private practice in Caboolture. There we built a new surgery; I had some wonderful experiences there and I expanded my knowledge of ADD and associated problems.

I eventually stated my own general practice in Kallangur, in that my interest in Child guidance and family practice our continued; side by side as it were with my general practice; I continued with my further training and interest in general and child psychiatry. I eventually retired from practice. I described the wonderful party that my patient put on for me. I found myself giving the much the same advice to the parents of children with problems; especially the children with ADHD; it convinced and made me more adamant to write this book. Along the way I did discuss many of treatment that have been proposed for ADHD; along the way I made some comments of other conditions such as Asperger's syndrome. I presented you with a developmental model, a discussion of the available **effective** treatments and I highlighted ineffective treatments. I suggested that maybe we should not consider ADHD not as a disease but a variant of normality. I discussed the many dramatic reports of the many ineffective treatments that have been suggested from time to time. I brought you the opinions of some fathers and I discussed the value of modeling that teaches better than word alone. Finally, I tried to emphasis; by my personal examples; that ADD is not a sentence and if it is well managed children grow up as successful adult. I am a doctor and I am sure that I had and probably still have some of the features of ADHD; maybe I could have been a specialist if effective treatments had have been available back then. It is important to encourage the interest and skills that any child has. There are very many successful individuals that have or had ADHD or Asperger's syndrome.

One of my ADD children grew up to have multiple degrees in computing and business his business has achieved Microsoft Gold accreditation. My other son is an A grade mechanic, runs his own business and has a very fruitful family life. My third son was a success and high earning salesman. My girls both have degrees and extremely successful in their respective careers. One has a degree in economics now is in enterprise banking; the other has several degrees in teaching and computing and presently directing infant schooling. I consider myself as a shining example that ADHD is not a life sentence.

ACKNOWLEDGEMENTS

To my valued teachers that got me ready for medicine and dealt with my ADD even before effective treatment was available.

To my University of Melbourne teachers, my early clinical teachers and my subsequent clinical teacher in Geelong hospital, and my teachers in Brisbane that introduced me to the subject that became my passion, ADD.

To the many teachers that were sponsored by the various drug companies that helped me get level 3 mental health accreditation.

www.ingramcontent.com/pod-product-compliance
Lightning Source LLC
Chambersburg PA
CBHW021419170526
45164CB00001B/20